ALL

ABOUT

ADDICTION

Ann Vitori,
RN, Ph.D.

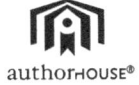

authorHOUSE®

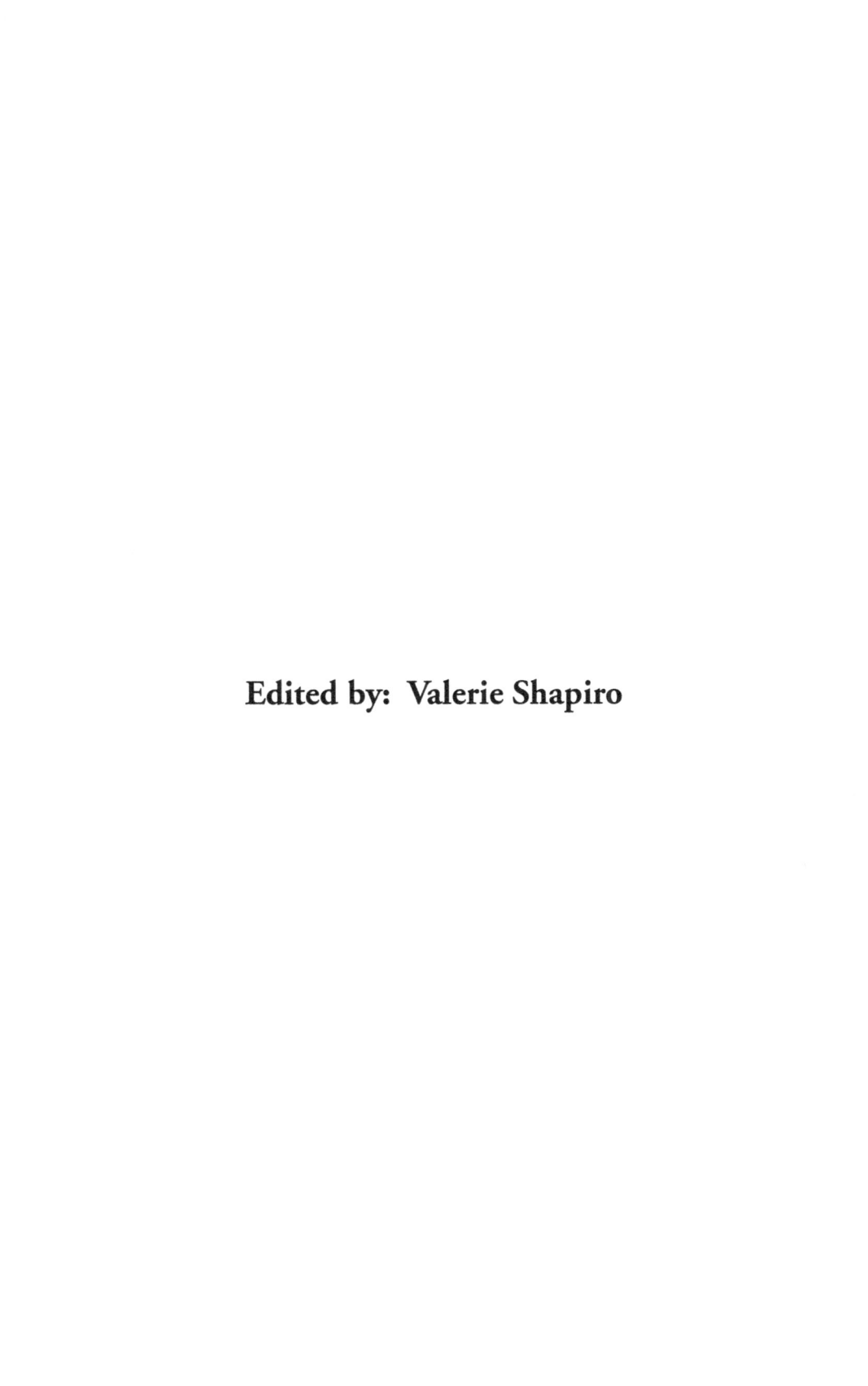

Edited by: Valerie Shapiro

AuthorHouse™
1663 Liberty Drive, Suite 200
Bloomington, IN 47403
www.authorhouse.com
Phone: 1-800-839-8640

First published by AuthorHouse 4/20/2009

ISBN: 978-1-4389-6839-1 (sc)

Printed in the United States of America
Bloomington, Indiana

This book is printed on acid-free paper.

DEDICATED

To my husband Frank, who encouraged me to write this book. Without his support and help, this would not have been written. Also, to my children, David, Valerie and Ronnie, for their assistance and contributions.

Table of Contents

INTRODUCTION:

There are many controversies regarding the causes of addiction. Many think it is genetics, mental illness, lack of willpower, poverty, moral weakness and anti-social personalities. Some believe it is a disease, although this theory lacks sufficient evidence.

People become addicted when they strive to fill some hole in their life because they feel a lack of love, acceptance, respect, recognition or acknowledgement. They try to fill this hole with drugs, alcohol, gambling, shopping, having sex with multiple partners and any other excessive behavior.

Pleasure is a very strong motivator for drug addiction. Opiate drugs attach to the receptor sites for pleasure but are much more potent than the natural opiates your brain produces. Once a person experiences this kind of pleasure, they crave more of it and their bodies build up a tolerance so it requires a stronger dose to get the same feeling. Stopping without professional help can be dangerous too. Once addicts realize they have a problem they may try to stop cold turkey. With drugs like Xanax, this can produce seizures. Medical detox centers can manage these symptoms as well as provide group and personal therapies. In order to stay free, addicts need the follow-up support from attending group therapies and AA or NA meetings. Many tragic deaths occur from patients who detox off of high doses and then have a relapse. When they use again, they will take the same dose they last took before detox., but now this dose is toxic to their body and they die.

No exact mechanism or gene has ever been identified but experts agree that some people are genetically vulnerable to addiction. Children of addicted parents are three to four times more likely to become addicts. However, this doesn't mean they are doomed to chemically dependent lives.

Some substances are more addictive than others due to the pharmacology of the substance and the mood of the user. Doctors who specialize in addiction have theorized that some people have deficiencies in their brain reward systems with fewer receptor sites and fewer circulating natural opiates. This condition may develop in early childhood with children who never learn to self-soothe when they are stressed. After years of abusing drugs, the addict desensitizes their receptors and ends up with altered pleasure thresholds. This is why it takes more and more of the drug to get the same effect.

People who are unhappy, with low self-esteem, no goals, no respect, can be easily influenced and vulnerable. They use substances to enhance or create pleasure in their lives, or to decrease the constant emotional pain they live with. Addicts self-medicate to feel normal. The better a person feels about himself, the less likely he will use or abuse any substances.

Hating their life and the feeling of rejection is how the potential addict is experiencing life. People want to be loved and accepted. Instead, they may be ridiculed and put down for many reasons, such as appearance, intelligence, race or social standing in the community.

A child faces rejection at an early age because they want to fit in. They could feel they are too tall, too small, too fat or skinny, not pretty or smart enough. Anxiety occurs from moving to a new place, going to a new school, or even traveling on vacations. Their parents may want them to go to college, but they feel they are non-achievers, and fear failure. Teens and young adults are particularly vulnerable because they are often unequipped to handle the strong emotions they feel from a negative event such as a break-up, divorce or death of a loved one. They would rather self-medicate and feel nothing than deal with their strong feelings of sadness or anger. Belonging and being part of a group, cult, and gang can also be very important to them. Peer pressure is extremely strong. They need to feel that they finally belong and have friends who accept and understand them.

There are proven methods for overcoming addiction based on studies and research.

We are familiar with Alcoholics Anonymous twelve-step program. There are values placed by the individual person, as to how important the addiction is, and the importance of things that will be lost to the addiction.

Many families break up due to addiction; parents who lose their jobs due to substance abuse, leave their children alone to feed their addiction, and make bad decisions while under the influence.

Our country depends on our youth to carry on, but, according to what is happening in our school districts, even as early as primary school, our students are introduced to drugs and alcohol. Many lives are lost due to overdoses and making bad decisions due to impaired brain function. Teenagers that have their entire future ahead of them are lost.

Healthy brain development is critical around the ages of 1-3. It is around this time that children learn to self-soothe when stressed. A nurturing parent can help them to internalize this process. But the days of a parent being home with the child are gone. Everyone wants or needs that additional income from the second job, when both parents are working. The nice home, status car, vacations etc. appear to be more important than staying home and raising the family. A parent being home when children come home from school, knowing whom their friends are and where they are going is no longer the norm. Children may want to talk to you about their day, but they come home to an empty house. What ever happened to the Sunday afternoon meals with the entire family where everyone talks about what is on their mind? Sunday was a family day. Now, very little time is spent together as a family. When a child wants to talk, or has a problem, no one is there for them. The child feels that he or she is no longer important, and that moment is lost. This is when they are vulnerable to trouble, which is waiting in the background.

The Following Information Will Touch On Addiction, and Some Of The Different Approaches Of Treatments.

We usually think of addiction as a disease that needs medical treatment, rehab, or a support group. Although many of these programs prove initially successful, few or no statistics are available to prove their long-term success. Surprisingly, some people do quit addictions on their own. We are told that is impossible to quit an addiction without use of other services, yet, it is done. Certain drugs stimulate certain parts of the brain, which causes that brain to become "hooked" on the drug. However, with strong motivation, you can fight your own addictions.

When the threats of smoking became publicized, many people who had smoked addictively quit in one day. They quit without any kind of support treatment. Many of our servicemen and women who return after war, quit their addiction to smoking or drugs because it is unacceptable to their families. It is now known that second and even third hand smoke has serious health consequences to the families and friends of smokers. One father quit after hugging his daughter and the third hand smoke still on his sweater triggered her asthma attack. Businesses want to hire non-smokers because they do not want second and third hand smoke in their buildings or offices. There is also less absenteeism in non-smoking environments.

Addiction is very powerful; you use it when you are unhappy or bored. You turn toward an addiction for pleasure, security and gratification. Addiction is changeable, and you can escape it by changing your attitudes and behavior. People use addiction to deal with life as a response to stress. It's easier for them to blame their addiction on something else, instead of overcoming and dealing their own feelings. People will accept that the addict can't help it unless they get medical treatment. You can seek help from traditional rehab treatments and twelve-step programs. Help is available in many forms, and there are barriers and steps you have to take. People in Alcoholics Anonymous do not consider it therapy but call it a self-help group.

Quitting: Before you can successfully quit addictions you need motivation. It helps to have support from people with strong values, such as parents, family, friends, and therapists. People with stable homes, higher education, community service and good work history can help get you over your addiction. They help you focus on what you may lose if you continue on your destructive way. You realize that you are not only hurting yourself, but also your family and friends.

You need to stop focusing on yourself, seek higher goals, commit yourself to helping others, think positively and be a positive contribution to the world. You are special, and remember, God made you, and he doesn't make junk.

A critical role, in addition, is your values. What is important to you? Refocus your thoughts to develop values. What is it that means everything to you?

Values come from your family, religion, education, background and cultural training. This starts when you are an infant, and grows as you grow and learn right from wrong and what is acceptable and non-acceptable behavior. Value your health, your home, your family and children. It's embarrassing to yourself and your family to be out of control in a drug or alcoholic stupor. You cannot help anyone else, fulfill your obligations, or succeed in school or business. What is more important to you? Being in control or giving in to your desires.

Values influence your ability to fight for what you believe in and care about.

There is no facilitator more important to fight addiction than your values. People with values want to be in control at all times, and will avoid intoxication of any kind. If you are concerned about your family, you will not allow yourself to drink excessively, poison your body with drugs, gamble, or engage in undiscriminating sex. Remember, when you are with many partners, it's as if you are having sex with everyone that your partner had before you. Who knows what disease or illness anyone had. Even with condoms, it is possible to pick up any number of diseases through oral or physical contact. Is your life or your spouse's life worth it? Your body is your temple and you should want to keep it clean and healthy.

It is a known fact that our outside jobs and positions influence our social values and personal factors.

Building blocks for living are what it takes to lead a full and satisfying life. Also, these same building blocks are needed to overcome addiction, whether on your own or through treatment. People can achieve remission by creating the fundamental building that form nonaddicted lives.

Basic Building Blocks:

Values   Support
Motivation   Mature Identity
Rewards   Goals
Resources

VALUES: The key to your escaping addiction. Consider what is important to you, sometimes refocusing on dormant values, or developing new ones. Your beliefs are that some things are right and others wrong. This is from your learning and background, your social and cultural group, training, religion and education. Children learn values from the people around them called social learning. Drinking is acceptable but socially governed, and people are taught to behave within clear boundaries, as to where, when and how much you can consume. Self-control, achievement, healthfulness, self-efficacy and responsibility are significant factors in controlling excess and addiction. You need to find your own values, and what factors in your life are important to you. Consider your family, friends, health, religious beliefs, profession, job, intelligence, appearance, respect for yourself and others.

MOTIVATION: People change when they want to change. It cannot be forced on them. Repeated failures are demoralizing and you may need to try something new. It also means that you are not in the right place in your life to change. Don't get down on yourself. Changes take different forms. Responsibility for changing your addictive behavior is up to you. You are a valuable person. What do you want for yourself? How are you going to achieve this? What is important to you? Why are you unable, or refusing to change your habit that is harming you?

REWARDS; People quit their addictions when they begin to get more rewards for living without them. In economic terms, your habit costs exceed its benefits. You incur many costs from an addiction, plus dangers to your health, financial, legal, interpersonal lives, just to name a few.

If you are unlucky to have been born with an intrinsic urge to drink, take drugs, or other addictions, perhaps your brain is wired in a way that these activities create impulses for you that need to be controlled. These excessive impulses provide you with feelings that you desire and want. It's a sense of being a worthwhile person. In time, addiction takes over and your life begins to revolve around it, and your indulgence becomes the first place you turn when unhappy or under stress.   You lose focus on how the addiction is damaging you, and take the sensations as rewards. To overcome any destructive habit, you have to get a handle on why you turn toward it. Only then you can identify how you can find superior nonaddictive rewards to take its place.

It is important to distinguish why you rely on addictions, perhaps to attain positive sensations like relaxation or to avoid negative feelings like anxiety and depression.   The first group uses addiction to feel good, and the latter group relies on it in order to cope with their emotions such as depression. People take it for granted that substance such as drugs are so pleasurable that it is almost impossible to resist them. The feeling of uncontrollable intoxication is not pleasurable for most people. While some found drugs enjoyable, they cannot function in a "high" state while they have to go about their busy days. They wanted to be in control of their own body. Most people find drugs less attractive and less important than making a living, supporting a family, and maintaining a position in society.

Family and work responsibilities are two most powerful experiences we have and this reward regularly outweighs the benefits provided by substance abuse.

Do not procrastinate or wait for a traumatic event, such as heart attack, diabetes, bankrupt or divorce. Think about the many catastrophic situations as reasons to fight addiction. Waiting to change can have serious drawbacks and may be too late. Thinking you can control your usage is an illusion. Once you are under the influence, you make poor decisions.

Here is an activity that may be helpful to clarify your goals. On a piece of paper, list all of the things that are most important to you. Prioritize your list and focus on the one thing that is the most important. Now write down all of the positive effects that letting go of your addiction will have on this one thing. Is the value of this worth the high you will be missing? Can you put another's needs above your own? You may be surprised by the different kind of high you derive from self-sacrifice. Can you love someone more than yourself? You will get back much more than you give. Now list the positive results for the rest of the items on your list. Can you see how valuable your recovery will be not only to yourself but those you love?

Once you have identified the reasons that you resort to the addiction, you can use less harmful replacements, which are known as
Replacement Alternatives.

1. Recognize, identify and focus on the negative consequences of your behavior
2. Reframe, recast a purposed reward of your behavior as a drawback
3. Replace a supposed benefit of the addiction with a less harmful alternative

Negatives Influences Causing your Life To Be Miserable.:
1. Divorce or breaking up of families / Extended families
2. Legal problems
3. Difficulties at work
4. Health problems
5. Disapproval of spouse, family, friends community
6. Financial problems, and loss of possessions
7. Self-esteem problems

Think how the costs and benefits have shifted. Think about the benefits of your addiction when it first began, and compare these to the benefits you now seek.

RESOURCES: To overcome addiction, evaluate your strengths and weaknesses and address your weaknesses effectively. Assess what resources you already have and what resources you currently lack. Develop the skills that will allow you to expand your resources. For example, during a break or after work, do you need substance, such as alcohol, smoking or drugs to relax, or would you be better off taking a walk, playing sports such as tennis, baseball, taking a shower etc. Even being able to afford treatment at rehab centers is no guarantee of overcoming substance abuse. Resources are not limited to money. For example:

1. Intimacy and supportive relationships, (for friendships, groups)
2. Employment and work resources, (work skills and accomplishments)
3. Leisure activities, hobbies and interests, ways of relaxing, exercise
4. Coping skills, practical & social, emotional resilience & ability to deal with stress.

You already possess the basic resources required to **Escaping Addiction**, and what ever destructive habit you may have. Identifying resources you already possess is a big part of the recovery process. The resources you now command give you confidence you have gained from you're past accomplishments, such as disadvantages, setbacks and crises you have overcome in your past already.

1. Look at your life? What resources do you have at your disposal, such as:
2. Good at repairing homes
3. Organized and smart with money
4. Friendly, well liked
5. Always able to get and hold a job

Good relationship with the community, family, friends, peers etc.

These resources will help you deal with stress.

Being gifted in the above area means you are closer to beating the addiction or negative behavior. Social skills enable you to deal with people, problem solve, and manage emotions that drive you to resort to addictions.

Essential skills for avoiding and **escaping addiction** are:

1. Communication,
2. Problem solving
3. Independence
4. Managing negative emotions
5. Resisting urges
6. Breaking the flow of destructive behavior.

Their negative outlooks characterize addicts; they experience life as a series of problems that they are unable to cope with. They panic and feel depressed due to their hopelessness and turn to addiction as a way to cope.

Template for coping with problems:

1. Identify the nature and scope of problem
2. Speak positively to yourself about your ability to cope
3. Identify specific steps to take to manage the challenge
4. Gather information and review options for responding
5. Relish your success at dealing with challenges.

You are most likely to turn to addictions when you are lonely and bored. You seek out company of others, even if they have a negative impact on your life. Addicts tag along with any group that will accept them, even if they indulge in destructive behavior to prove membership in the group.

You need to learn how to spend time by yourself constructively without desperation. This requires skills or resources, such as being able to enjoy time alone, to self soothe, rather than look to other people to calm you. You can achieve calmness by yoga, meditation, walking, exercising reading, television viewing, hobbies, writing etc. As you develop basic life resources, you will be more able to spend time alone. Picture yourself as a respectable responsible person that you can look at with pride.

You will need to find new outlets for venting your feelings and anger constructively. What kind of negative emotions are still limiting your recovery process? The longer you practice your new approach to managing your emotions, the more effective this process will become. Your coping skills will grow as you practice your ability to deal with yourself in situations.

Dealing With Emotional Upset:

1. Identify situations that trigger angry, depressed, or bored feelings, and avoid such situations.
2. Reframe these events to defuse your emotional reactions to them and change how you view and label an event.
3. Use a relaxation technique to delay or avoid an emotional reaction by counting to 10 or leaving the room (if permitted).

4. Develop and review techniques for addressing your upset, such as speaking clearly and unemotionally to the person upsetting you.
5. Find a technique to help when a person you deal with regularly is the source of the upset. Ask the person please not to act that way in the future. Stay away from the upsetting person or provocative situation.

There are ways to resist addictive urges and are classified as Cognitive, Behavioral and Social.

Your Power In Fighting Addiction:

Cognitive – Make a list of the positive consequences of quitting the behavior and the negative consequences of continuing it.

Behavioral – substitute eating or drinking something healthy, physical activity, exercise, relaxation, select a distracting activity or delaying activity.

Social - seeking social support, escaping the situation

It is important to recognize your own power in fighting addiction. You must recognize you have the ability to immediately regain control after a slip. Whenever you feel yourself sliding out of control, remember that you have a choice. If you wish to escape, then you can pull yourself out of the problem. You can always make your problem worse. That is why you should stop NOW. You have already done damage to your health, and its time to give your body a break. You have already caused pain to loved ones, but you still have options available to you. You must take responsibility for your actions. You have the ability to apply the brakes. You need to know how to communicate and ask for help to deal with negative emotions. Your family and friends will always love you and will appreciate your confidence in their ability to help.

SUPPORT: Our associations with parents and peer groups influence how we respond (either positively or negatively) to certain situations. This is true about drugs, alcohol, food etc. All of us must learn the skills of moderate consumption. Like we all say, "Everything in moderation." Social learning of addictive behaviors involves factors that make an individual more or less likely to be overwhelmed by negative behavior. Some factors that lead to unhealthy addictive substance use are:

1. The individual is not part of a responsible social group or stable setting
2. The individual uses a substance either in isolation or with people who do not or can not care for them
3. The user is introduced to the substance by people who are addicts
4. Use of the substance is an excuse for antisocial, irresponsible or uncontrolled behavior.

Maturity Identity:

Children raised in households where substance such as alcohol and drugs are abused may find it difficult not to abuse this substance themselves.

Children in a family where drinking is absent can face similar difficulties. In this case, no social learning takes place because drinking is considered dangerous and unmanageable. Further more, they learn these habits from, high school peers, fellow college students, or the military. They are without a support network of moderate drinkers.

You can join a twelve-step group, such as AA, a group of former drinkers, NA, Gamblers Anonymous, Sex Addicts Anonymous, Shoppers Anonymous, Overeaters Anonymous etc. These self-help groups are groups that individuals join to find support from others, rather than go it alone.

Other alternative groups are Smart Recovery, and Moderation Management.

Also, spouses can join Al-Anon or your children can join Alateen. Family members are taught the same thing addicts learn in AA. With this support, you are always going to meetings. The group socializes and enjoys many experiences in life without partying.

Another option is to form your own group among people you know that have needs similar to yours. Many people exercise together, rides bikes walk with friend's etc. Spend time with people you already know, whose goals and expectations are similar to your own.

The best strategy is to create your own small culture of health and responsibility at home, or elsewhere. You can succeed in modifying your own thinking, behavior, social reality and the course of your life. Think of a few people you know whose behavior you admire or want to emulate. Spend time with them, engaging in the behavior you want to change. Ask them for suggestons, which is called coaching. They will become part of your change support group.

MATURE IDENTITY: Immature gratification is the search of self-seeking behavior resembling that of a dependent child. This phenomenon is known as maturing out. The individual outgrows their addiction, they are tired of being on the outside, cut off from normal life, constant hustling and evading the law, wanting a better life, good job, family and respect of others. As you mature, you become dissatisfied with what you have not accomplished. You need a positive identity, need new behavior, a self-image or identity to be proud of.

Addiction is a childlike search for constant security and gratification. It is a vocation that will wrap its life around the addict. The life of an addict is a series of stealing, even from family and friends, plus assuring the connection of his or her supplier and staying one step ahead of the police. Performing the rituals of preparing and taking the substance is a vocation around which the addict builds his or her life.

As the addict gets older, he or she begins to see what they are missing, a full life, family, and a job. They recognize the costs of their addiction, being known as a tramp, slut, bum, and loser. The social pressure becomes harder and harder. They cannot stay healthy and live. They start to eat less and drink less, they bodies no longer can tolerate excess. They do not have the disposable income to support expensive habits. Then, you start to gain faith in yourself, change the way you experience and react to different events in your life. As you mature, you are more able to control your reactions or over reactions, you are less likely to need to resort to addictive remedies.

Growing into maturity means focusing less on your weaknesses and non-abilities and more on your responsibilities to yourself and to others.

You need to take responsibility for your addiction. It used to be that drugs were considered irresistible, but today, that is not the case. Individuals can stop addictions just as they can stop eating potato chips and food that is dangerous to their health. They need to accept responsibilities for their habits.

After years of detox and rehab, the individual must take responsibility of his actions and liberate from the addiction. You have the power to attack the addiction, You can free yourself. Fulfill your obligation to yourself. Its failure to assume that your addiction forces you to behave in a negative fashion, not caring about anything or anybody and resorting to theft to support your habit.

Examine yourself and your life. Understand the nature of maturity and how it overcomes addiction. Strive to develop the qualities of maturity.

1. Develop the tools and experience you acquired. You will be able to accomplish necessary and worthwhile things.
2. Recognize the good you have done and also be more realistic about yourself and your accomplishments.
3. Be tolerant of others, people are who they are, take the good with the bad.

4. Take responsibility for your actions and behavior.

5. You have obligations. Others are counting on you.

6. Have faith, you will survive this.

There are people who overcame addictions during the course of their lives without treatment. Self-curers often cure their addiction consciously themselves. These individuals broke free and did not need to unlearn the destructive labels that treatment sometimes impose on them.

Only the mature adult with self-determination will make this choice of freedom from addiction. They want to reclaim their dignity and lead productive lives. Leading a new life, not calling attention to your addiction and not visualizing your addiction in every situation are parts of developing your new identity.

The non-addict self image will bolster your new self-view. They leave behind their addiction which controlled their lives and proudly lead lives that are consistent with their values which others admired. They are secure and in control of their bodies at all time. They always know what they are doing. They have become assets in their community.

GOALS: When a habit or addiction interferes with accomplishing a goal you want to attain, you are inclined to quit. It is critical to focus on what you want to achieve, not quit and give up for your addiction, Worthwhile personal goals are those you pursue to make yourself a better person. Setting self-improving goals and the steps necessary to achieve them include exercising and pursuing your education or other training. Advancing your career, maintaining and improving relations in your family are also things that contribute to a constructive and happy life.

Personal Life Goals:

Family- Enjoy home life, spend time with family, create a positive home atmosphere and take an interest in your family's activities an thoughts.

Work – Take pride in your work. Focus on your job and go above and   beyond your job description. Work hard to impress the boss, and maybe you'll get a promotion.

Health- Maintain a healthy weight to improve health, jog or walk four days a week, join a gym, eat healthy meals and snacks.

Addiction-Stop indulging in your addiction, come home right after work, feel good about work and your family, think positively about yourself.

These are goals needed to fight addiction. They make you feel better about yourself and to have control over activities in your life that matter. Addicts focus exclusively on their own needs and are insufficiently connected emotionally with the world and lives of people around them. Lack of concern and behaving selfishly while the addict pursues their addiction is a powerful reason to quit.

Addicts disregard the well being of others. They make poor decisions and exhibit inappropriate behaviors. For example, they are noisy, intoxicated, irresponsible, litter with cigarette butts, steal, become violent, are poor role models for children, cost society for health care and are unable to contribute to others or society.

Some family and individual problems that are factors for addiction are family alcohol usage, poor inconsistent family management practices, intense family conflict, poor bonding, early problem behavior, academic failure, peer rejection, association with substance users, rebellious, and poor attitudes regarding family and community.

Pursuing goals are beneficial. What good things do you do for yourself, for your family? How does this make you feel? What contribution have you made to society and how did this make you feel?

We need to recognize the larger goals implicated in the fight against addiction.

TREATMENT:
Managed Care: Over 45 million Americans do not have health insurance. 43% of people who seek treatment, cite no insurance coverage as the main reason for not getting it. Even with coverage, some insurance companies do not allow the treatment facilities to give the necessary treatments for the proper length of time. We need to build a better system. We need to make treatment programs available to everyone that needs them regardless of insurance status. Programs must provide needed skills that enlist people's values and motivations without labeling them. All addiction counselors should learn how to provide skills training and motivations. Treatments should be coordinated with services and family support, housing, job training, medi-

cal care, and psychotherapy for other emotional problems. Focus needs to be on addicts as they live, experience, and react to the world and treatment must include follow-up. We need to have policies and programs that improve addict's lives including training on how to get and hold a job, maintain their health, stabilize their family and home lives, reduce criminal activity and remove the stigma of being an addict.

We will never find a single magical cure for addiction, as though it were located somewhere in the brain. Instead, addiction will be reduced only in a better world comprised of better-equipped people leading better lives.

The first medical breakthrough in treatment was the discovery of Methadone in the 60s to combat heroine addiction. Now, for people determined to overcome opiate addiction, suboxone has proven to be an effective tool. Research is ongoing to find new and effective medications to help in recovery.

The American foreign policy cannot continue to be dominated by anti-drug mania. We spend millions of dollars to eradicate crops, support regimes that promise to suppress the drug trade etc. But it is not working. We need more focus on education, prevention and treatment here at home. Rehab programs must be regulated, government subsidized, results based and readily available to all who want to attend regardless of their ability to pay. Rehab programs should be accountable for their results and maintain funding by certifying positive results and maintaining patient follow-up.

ALCOHOL:

Ethanol or ethyl alcohol is a sedative-hypnotic drug that acts on the human brain like other sedative-hypnotic drugs. This can cause physical dependence in anyone who consumes enough of it for a sufficient period of time. Withdrawal syndrome is identical to that of other drugs in the same class such as Valium, Librium, Xana, Ativan, and other barbiturates. Regular exposure to any of these may develop the following symptoms upon abrupt discontinuation or drastic reduction of dosage:

> Anxiety, restlessness, irritability, insomnia, elevated blood pressure, temperature, pulse and respiration; Confusion, hypervigilance and disorientation, visual and auditory hallucinations, acute psychotic behavior, grand mal seizures infrequently sudden death.

These symptoms from alcohol will develop in anyone exposed to it long enough, regularly enough and in sufficient dosage if intake is suddenly curtailed. The addict cannot really and truly desire recovery until he is ready for it. Specific behavior that characterizes alcoholism is the consumption of significant quantities of alcohol on repeated occasions. They have this craving or compulsion to drink. Symptoms associated with depression and anxiety disorder, such as insomnia, low mood, irritability, chest pain, palpitations, dyspnea often occur. Alcohol seems to relieve these symptoms, resulting in a vicious cycle of drinking followed by depression, then by drinking etc. Many alcoholics find abstinence from alcohol difficult or impossible to achieve or to maintain. The addicts mind is no longer his mind but has become an agent and tool of the addiction. Recovery is recovery of life itself, getting back something of value, not giving up something that is strongly desired. Addiction is a form of bondage.

The craving and mental obsession of the alcoholic causes then to drink repeatedly, and causes problems for themselves, their family, friends and others.

INTERVENTION of the alcoholic consists of family, friends, co-workers, and others. expressing their concern. This is the gateway from a deteriorating existence to a healthy and rewarding sobriety.

Obstacles to recovery from addiction are shame, dishonesty, ignorance and the alcoholic's personal beliefs that he can overcome this anytime he wants.

Going into recovery for the addict is like exploring a frightening unknown place without maps, guides or landmarks. Words idea theories etc can take you just so far, but they are enough to guide the addict through their own trial and error tactics. It's like riding a bicycle, falling off, and getting back on. The struggle to make it balance and go where they want to go is worth all the obstacles and resistance.

Like a malignant tumor, addiction invades and destroys the body. Time is required for this process to develop, and, time is required for a tumor to spread and infiltrate healthy issue. The longer the process has been underway, the more difficult it is to halt or reverse it.

Addiction behavior attempts to repair a state of bad feeling, and can be compared to an unhealthy love affair. Recovery is restoring natural and healthy regulation of mood and feelings. Because addicts may be seriously impaired in their pre-addictive self-care, they often require prolonged help learning to feel well without addiction.

Although the treatment for alcoholism is just don't drink the alcohol. It seems like a simple theory, but, it is not easy in practice for individuals with the illness of alcohol dependence.

Instead of telling the alcoholic they are ruining their life, tell them how many times they called in sick, and how many times they were in a drunken state, and how much money they are spending. Make sure they know you love and will support them. Do not give in. Treat them with respect and dignity, but do not condone their behavior. Tough love is a way to go.

Once a person is determined to get well, there are some medications that can help. Disulfiram (Antabuse) will produce acute sensitivity to alcohol and give severe symptoms of a hangover in 5 to 10 minutes after a drink. Other medications like Acamprosate (Canpral) and Naltrexone (Revia, Depade) can reduce your desire for alcohol once you stop drinking.

TEENAGE BINGE DRINKING:

Alcohol use in teens and preteens is on the rise. Binge drinking used to mean drinking heavily over a period of several days. Today, it's the consumption of five or more drinks in a row. College students seem to be most susceptible to binge drinking. They are out of the house, living on their own, going to parties where alcohol is easily accessible. Peer pressure is the most common reason for drinking. They want to be accepted and popular. Binge drinking can have life threatening consequences. When someone drinks too much at one time, they can get alcohol poisoning that affects the body's involuntary reflexes of breathing. Also, a person can choke to death on his or her vomit. Other symptoms include confusion, vomiting, seizures and irregular breathing. Binge drinking also impairs your judgment. The teen may drink and drive, have unprotected sex, and may be a target for assault or rape. Binge drinking may cause frequent waking at night and a change in attitude or grades. Communication is key. Parents can help influence their child's beliefs about positive or negative effects of drinking.

Peer pressure is very real and very strong. Everyone wants to be accepted; to be part of the group. Teens will go against what their parents say, what they have been taught during the years, just to belong, to be cool, to be one of the group. In the group, they are never alone, and feel they are someone special, will always have someone who cares.

This also makes them vulnerable to brainwashing by cults. They are told the cult is their family, and they care about them.

DRUG ABUSE:

Drug abuse, prescription drugs and street drugs involve the repeated and excessive use of drugs, prescription or street drugs. Almost all drugs over stimulate the pleasure center of the brain, flooding it with neurotransmitter dopamine, which produces euphoria. These drugs increase energy, rapid heart rate and elevated blood pressure. Continued use causes rapid breathing, irritability, impulsiveness, aggression, nervousness, insomnia, weight loss, tolerance, addiction, and possible heart failure. They also cause impairment; cognitive functioning which negatively affects memory and impacts the ability to learn.

SIGNS AND SYMPTOMS OF DRUG ABUSE:
1. Continuing to use drugs even though you no longer have problems
2. Irritability, anger, hostility, fatigue, agitation, anxiety, depression, Psychosis, difficulty concentrating
3. Paying bills late, inability to keep track of your money
4. Being arrested, doing things that you normally do not do, stealing

5. Missing work or school, being late due to drug use
6. Annoyed when criticize about using drugs
7. Associating with questionable acquaintances to purchase drugs
8. Schedule your day around using drugs
9. Focusing recreational activities around obtaining and using drugs
10. Heightened visual and auditory perceptions, sensitivity to taste
11. Problems with memory, difficulty concentrating, paranoid thinking
12. Decreased coordination slowed reaction time.

People with Attention-Deficit/Hyperactivity Disorder, depression and anxiety may find that a street drug makes them feel less jumpy or anxious.

Drugs become priority, and you are willing to sacrifice your work, home and family. As your brain and body build a tolerance to the substance, you begin to require larger and more frequent doses in order to achieve the same effect.

The severity of withdrawal symptoms such as shakes, muscle pain, nausea, vomiting, headaches, cravings can be reduced in detox with prescribed medications that can be slowly decreased over time.

SHORT TERM EFFECTS OF HEROIN:
Rush, depressed respiration, clouded mental function, nausea and vomiting, suppression of pain.

LONG TERM EFFECTS OF HEROIN:

Infectious diseases (HIV/AIDS/Hepatitis), collapsed veins, bacterial infections, abscesses, infection of heart lining and valves, arthritis and other rheumaatologic problems.

<u>COMMONLY ABUSED DRUGS;</u>

Cocaine – Ritalin – Ecstasy – Heroin – Vicodin and Oxycontin – Valium, Soma and Xanax – Marijuana and Hashish – Magic Mushrooms – LSD and PCP – Aerosols, Nitrous Oxide, Nitrites (poppers) – Anabolic steroids.

An aspirin a day has gained the reputation of being essential to good health.

The key lies in knowing which dose is best. Aspirin helps prevent the formation of heart attack and stroke causing blood clots, but, it increases the risk of bleeding. Aspirin in the stomach exerts the effect to weaken the barrier between the stomach's tissues and causing gastric acids, which may lead to fatal ulcers. It is also linked to hemorrhage stroke, which occurs when the wall of a weakened blood vessel burst. Some teens start taking aspirin in high doses for a high.

The good news in the war on drugs is that the United States is making progress in beating back the availability of drugs like cocaine and methamphetamines. The bad news is the emerging drugs of choice come straight out of the family medicine cabinet. Prescription drugs are the new gateway drugs for the new generation of addicts. Teens and addicts now turn to prescription drugs, painkillers and tranquilizers that are accessible and comparably cheap. Nevertheless, they are addictive and damage lives just as street drugs. 60

percent of prescription drug abusers get their supply from relatives or friends for free.

Throw out unused prescriptions that you no longer need, so teens on the prowl are not tempted to take them.

COMMON WARNINGS OF TEEN DRUG USE:

1. Poor school performance, declining grades, increased absences, truancy
2. Withdrawal from hobbies, teams, family life
3. Marked change in behavior ranging from hostility to violence
4. Changes in energy level, such as unusual amounts of energy, or fatigue
5. Increased secrecy about possessions or activities
6. Use of incense, room freshener, perfume
7. Wearing new clothes that highlight drug use, inappropriate conduct
or lack of concern for appearance and grooming
8. Evidence of drug paraphernalia, pipes and rolling papers
9. Missing prescription drugs
10. Unusual requests for money without reasonable explanations.
Discovering money stolen from your home or purse, or, discovering objects missing which may have been stolen.

Young ER patients with heart attack symptoms should be asked if they have recently used cocaine, which can cause similar chest pain. Some heart attack treatments can be deadly to someone using cocaine. Not knowing what you are dealing with and giving the wrong therapies could mean death rather than benefit.

<u>ANOTHER THREAT TO OUR YOUTH;</u>

A new threat has been emerging called cheese. This "cheese" is a concoction of Mexican black-tar heroin and crushed medicine that contain antihistamine diphenhydrame, and sleep aids. When cheese is combined with the effects of heroin, you get a double whammy to your body, two downers at once. When mixed together, it resembles grated Parmesan cheese, and it can kill you. The drug dealers are targeting middle schools kids and they are getting hooked on the snortable high. Middle school youth already struggle with peer pressure but now, it could kill them. Cheese is dangerous, and is very cheap. It can be snorted with a straw. Its symptoms include drowsiness, sluggishness, euphoria, excessive thirst, and disorientation.

The danger is very real. It takes over your body and start slowing everything inside down, eventually slowing down the heart until it stops and you are dead.

Cheese had its origin in Texas, where at least 21 youths have died from it and hundreds have been admitted to treatment facilities. (The full article can be read in the Tampa Tribune, Monday, Nov. 12, 2007 issue.)

Abusing drugs destroys your life, your memory, your self-respect, and everything that is connected with your self-esteem. Recreational drugs never helped anybody. Inappropriate use of drugs can harm or even kill you.

You may be hooked emotionally and psychologically. You may have a physical dependence too. If you have a drug addiction, whether legal or illegal drug, you have intense cravings for it. You want to use the drug again and again. When you stop taking it, you have unpleasant physical reactions.

Breaking a drug addiction is difficult, but not impossible. Support from your doctor, family, friends, and others will help you beat your drug dependence.

Communities need to educate youth on the extreme danger of "Cheese" and other drugs.

In working with young drug abusers, two issues must be realized:
1. Drugs are a waste of time, they destroy your life, memory, self respect and self-esteem
2. Drugs never helped anybody study better, play sports better, sing better play music better or do anything better, but, they can kill you

Treatment options are the decision of the addict as to what treatment programs, rehab, peer support groups and willpower that make him feel most comfortable. With new ways of coping with problems, without the use of drugs, the tight grip of addiction will began to loosen its hold. Recovery is possible with medical and social support.

FOOD ADDICTION:

This is a term used to describe a pathological disorder, compulsive, excessive craving for food. Only recently has there been an acceptance of the fact that persons may be addicted to food in the same way as they are addicted to alcohol or drugs. Any substance taken into the body regardless of its potential for harm or in excess is said to be abused.

Are you addicted? Ask yourselves a few key questions:

1. Do you eat when you are not hungry, or when depressed
2. Do you eat in secret, or differently when alone
3. Do you consume large amounts of food, then purge later by vomiting or using laxatives
4. Are there foods you know are harmful to you, but eat them anyway
5. Do you feel guilty after eating

If you answer" yes" to any of these questions, you are likely to be addicted to food.

As with any addiction, food addiction is loss of control. You know the way you are eating is harmful, but continue the destructive behavior.

Some individuals have food allergies. Certain trigger foods when ingested cause negative symptoms, and at the same time provoke cravings. For example, the diabetic may become sick by ingesting sugar, but still continue to crave it and eat it in excess with adverse effects. Studies are continuing regarding certain proteins in milk and wheat which, when ingested, produce narcotic-like effects. These chemicals mimic the body's natural painkillers, endorphins. Individuals may be suffering from depression, low self-esteem or loneliness, and find a high when ingesting large quantities of certain foods such as salt, chocolate, or cheesecake. The immediate high gives way to a sick feeling or guilt leading to more depression. The addict is out of control and will again turn to the same eating patterns in an effort to feel better.

Food addiction is a disease characterized by obsession with weight and body image, and comes from all ages, race, gender and groups. They are overweight, underweight, and normal weight. The obese person suffers humiliation due to excess weight. He may be lethargic and sedentary unable to move around freely. The underweight person may be bulimic though they eat obsessively. They are afraid of becoming overweight and will induce vomiting, take laxatives, or exercise compulsively to prevent weight gain. The person with normal weight may be obsessed with food, constantly thinking what to eat or how much they weigh. The subject of food is a misery to them, and they count calories compulsively.

<u>Food addiction is similar to drug and alcohol addiction,</u> and is a serious condition with many adverse consequences such as obesity, psychological disorders, diabetes and gastric anomalies. For a food addict, refined sugar, flour and fats become what alcohol is to the alcoholic or cocaine to the cocaine addict.

The first step is realization and acceptance of the problem. First, the individuals must identify their trigger foods which cause allergic symptoms and cravings.

There is no easy way to combat food addiction. It requires intense discipline in modifying eating patterns and life-style. You will need a manageable exercise program along with dietary changes.

The physiological and psychological dependency of food can best be broken when the individual recognizes they are powerless to combat it alone.

Food addiction is characterized by:

1. Obsession - obsessed by the recalled sense of pleasure from a comfort food
2. Lack of self-control – Repeated use of this food can create pleasure and Comfort
3. Preoccupation – Preoccupied with finding sources of food associated with pleasure and comfort
4. Compulsion – Eating results in a cycle of bingeing despite knowledge of negative consequences

5. Craving – Although one can restrain oneself from eating, physical cravings can negate the power to make this decision

Binge eaters also have eating disorders, and are unable to control their food intake and attempts to lose weight by dieting. While there may be some weight loss, it is gained back as well as additional pounds. Binge eaters find that their eating or weight interferes with their relationship, their work and self –esteem. They give up dieting efforts and become depressed and anxious.

BULIMIA NERVOSA: purging, a potentially devastating disease, which are periods of binge eating. The binge eater consumes large amounts of food in a short period of time. They prevent weight gain by self-induced vomiting, laxative use or diuretics, compulsive exercising or misuse of insulin, if the bulimic is diabetic. They exhibit depression, irritability and severe mood swings.

ANOREXIA NERVOSA: It is a progressive and potentially fatal disease characterized by a 15% below normal body weight. Anorexic have an intense fear of fat and claims of feeling fat when they are very underweight.

Anorexics have trouble experiencing feelings or handling stressful situation in their lives. Restricting food becomes a way to numb their thoughts and feelings and establish a sense of power and control.

TREATMENT can work. Individuals realize after years of failed attempts that diets or starvation do not work and that professional help is needed to deal with their feelings of anger, fear and depression.

The most successful treatment treats the total person. Each person is unique and a plan is designed to meet his or her specific needs. Goals of treatment consist of:

1. Restoring healthy eating pattern and healthy body weight
2. Identifying and treating emotional issues that trigger symptoms
3. Developing coping strategies that will assist the individual in dealing with day to day stresses
4. Continuing support for long-term recovery

Obesity Consequences:

For a successful recovery, each individual should be provided with an education program consisting of lectures and workshops, individual therapy with a psychotherapist to help them regain control of their life, group therapy, and support groups to learn they are not alone.

The health consequences of obesity are tremendous. Many of our children now display atherosclerosis , which are fat deposits in the arteries leading to death from coronary artery disease. Large numbers of children are developing type 2 diabetes because of their lifestyle. An article in the Journal of American Medical Association states that the culprits in fattening American children are fast foods, soda, and junk foods found in schools and homes. Many parents work to give their children lunch money;   However,   the children buy burgers, french fries, candy, sweets, deserts and other garbage food. Also, they spend their recreational time sitting in front of electronic entertainment, such as television, video games and listening to music. They no longer engage in outdoor physical activities.

As with all substance abuse, the family tends to gain an understanding of the disease and recovery process. Recovery, to be successful, needs family, friends and co-workers working together, being non-judgmental. Also, working in a group with peers has proven very successful. Spirituality helps each person explore his or her relationship with a higher power. There are many sources of strength in recovery such as the twelve steps, philosophies of Overeaters Anonymous and Food Addict Anonymous. These are helpful models to utilize on this spiritual journey. This non-denominational journey into spirituality helps to realize there are many sources of strength in recovery.

Picture yourself as you want to look, set a goal, and work with diet and exercise to help achieve your goal.

GAMBLING:

Gambling is a progressive disease; it begins slowly and grows until the victim's life becomes progressively unmanageable. You cannot look at a person and detect by a breath test or blood test, that they have a gambling problem. Gambling does not leave needle marks.

Pathological gamblers hide their lottery tickets, sports picks, etc. from family, friends and co-workers. Gambling can be a means of escaping from problems in a marriage, work or within the family. Pathological gambling is known as a disorder of impulse control.

There are six types of gamblers:

1. Professional gamblers
2. Anti-social or personality gamblers
3. Casual social gamblers
4. Serious social gamblers
5. Relief and escape gamblers
6. Compulsive gamblers

Gamblers no longer need to go to Las Vegas or Atlantic City to find the action they crave. It is available in many of their own hometowns.

Legalized gambling is one of the fastest growing industries in the United States. We have off-track betting parlors (OTB), riverboat casinos, etc.

For most people, gambling is fun and a form of entertainment. However, it can be a devastating illness that affects every aspect of individual lives. It can be defined as playing a game of chance for stakes. Gambling occurs in many forms, such as horse and dog tracks, off-track-betting parlors, jai alai, lotteries, casinos, bookmaking, card rooms, bingo and the stock market.

Research indicates that adolescents are about three times more likely than adults to become problem gamblers. This sounds an alarm for the future and indicates a growing need for additional adult and adolescent gambling treatment counselors across the nation.

Warning Signs, which may indicate the individual has a gambling problem, especially in the work- place:

1. Excessive use of telephones, (to call bookmakers, stockbrokers or to obtain credit
2. Taking the company vehicle to the race track, card room, casino, etc. (parking tickets near gambling or racetrack locations are a red flag)
3. Absence from work, often for part of the day (typically after lunch)

4. Arriving late for work (related to all-night card games, casino trips, anxiety-related sleep disturbances)
5. Vacation days taken on isolated days rather than in weeks (or vacations to gambling locations on a regular basis
6. Sick days taken immediately or ahead of time
7. Failure to take days off (obsessed with getting money to pay gambling debts or afraid to take a day off because of fear that embezzlement or fraud will be discovered in their absence)
8. Changes in productivity (which seem to be related to mood swings)
9. Organizing office pools and gambling junkets
10.Borrowing money from co-workers or arguing with co-workers over failure to pay debts
11. Embezzlement, defrauding customers or engaging in employee theft for resale

The life of the compulsive gambler begins to fall apart as repeated efforts to gain control over their addiction fail. All compulsive gamblers can stop gambling for a while, but most people need professional help to stop.

If the compulsive gambler could stop chasing losses, he would. All compulsive gamblers can stop gambling for a while. However, most need professional help to stop for life.

There are recovery programs through the help of an outpatient rehabilitation program. This type of program does not require addicts to take time off from work, leave their families or enter a hospital as an inpatient. They involve a series of meetings four nights a week, with lectures and group therapy, on the order of the twelve-step programs of AA.

The progression of gambling addiction is known to include three phases:

The winning phase
The losing phase
And the desperation phase.

<u>The Winning Phase</u> - gamblers experience a big win or a series of wins that leaves them with unreasonable optimism that their winning will continue. They feel excitement when gambling and begin increasing the amounts of their bets.

<u>The Losing Phase</u> – gamblers often begin bragging about wins they had, start gambling alone, think more about gambling and borrow money, legally or illegally. They start lying to family and friends and become more irritable, restless and withdrawn. Their home life becomes unhappy, and they are unable to pay their bills. The gamblers begin to chase their losses, believing they must return as soon as possible to win back their losses.

<u>The Desperation Phase</u> – there is a marked increase in the time spent gambling, accompanied by remorse, blaming others and alienating family and friends. The gamblers may engage in illegal acts to finance their gambling. They experience hopelessness, suicidal thoughts and attempts, arrests, divorce, alcohol, drug abuse, or an emotional breakdown.

It is estimated that three percent of the adult population will experience serious problems with gambling that will result in significant debt, family disruption, job losses, criminal activity or suicide.

Pathological gambling affects gamblers, their families, their employers and the community. During phases of their addiction, they spend less time with their family and more of their family's money on gambling until their bank accounts are depleted. Eventually, they steal money from family members.

At work, the gambler miss-uses time in order to gamble, has difficulty concentrating and finishing projects, may engage in embezzlement, theft or other illegal activities.

SEX ADDICTION

Programs that focus on abstinence have not had any affect on teenager's sexual behavior. Presently, evidence fails to show that any abstinence program delays the initiation of sex, or reduce the number of sexual partners among teenagers.

The report is based on research into teen sexual behavior and released by the nonpartisan National Campaign to prevent teen and unplanned pregnancy. Abstinence appears to have little impact on the teens. Comprehensive sex education programs were having more positive outcomes, such as delaying initiation of sex, reducing the frequency, reducing the number of sexual partners, and increasing use of condoms. A study sought to debunk what the report called myths propagated by abstinence-only advocates. These myths claim that sex education promotes promiscuity and hastens the initiation of sex sending confusing message to the adolescent. None of these was found to be accurate.

Sex addiction involves a wide variety of practices. Sometimes an addict has trouble with one unwanted behavior, sometime more. Many sex addicts state their unhealthy use of sex has been a progressive process. It may have started with an addiction to masturbation, pornography, or a relationship, but over the years progressed to dangerous behaviors.

The essence of all addiction is the addict's experience of powerlessness over a compulsive behavior which causes their lives to becoming unmanageable. The addict is out of control, experiences tremendous shame, pain and self-loathing. The addict wants to stop, but fails to do so. Consequently, addicts suffer from losing relationships, difficulties with work, arrests, financial troubles, loss of interest in things not sexual, low self-esteem and despair. Preoccupation with sex takes up a great amount of energy. As this increases, the sex addict's pattern of behavior follows, which usually leads to acting out, flirting, driving to the park. When the acting out happens, there is a denial of feelings, usually followed by despair and shame or a feeling of hopelessness and confusion.

SEX - Offenders Behavior:

In its simplest form sex addiction is a normal sex drive that has become obsessive to the point that behavior is out of control. The euphoric feeling or high comes from chemicals released into the brain rather than from an external source. Sex addiction can take on many forms, from the use of pornography and masturbation to repeated affairs, patronizing prostitutes. In extreme cases, sex addiction can involve molestation, rape and murder. Sex addicts have one thing in common: the behavior is done in secret, and the sex addict becomes adept at hiding this secret from his family and friends.

It is rarely caused by only one factor, but more likely a build up of conditions over time. For some, the sex addiction can be triggered by traumatic experiences in their childhood, sexual abuse, abandonment, or emotional trauma. One of the most serious problems with sexual addiction is the way it affects relationships. Closeness in a marriage is a commitment. Relationships are comprised of physical, emotional, and spiritual aspects of the relationship. When one aspect starts to break down, the others tend to suffer as well. Sexual addiction is all about selfishness. The sex addict becomes obsessed with meeting his own needs at the expense of his partner.

For some sex addicts, behavior does not go beyond compulsive masturbation, pornography, phone, computer or sex service. Other addicts get involve in illegal activities such as exhibitionism, obscene calls, child molestation, and rape.

Sex offenders act out of a disturbed need for power, dominance, control or revenge. A sex addict will continue to engage in certain sexual behaviors despite facing potential health risks, financial problems, shattered relationships or arrest.

Like eating, having sex is necessary for human survival. Although some people are celibate, some not by choice, others choose celibacy for cultural or religious reasons. Healthy humans have a strong desire for sex, and lack of interest or low interest can indicate a medical problem or psychiatric illness.

SMOKING ADDICTION:

We hear quite a bit about smoking, and it appeared to be an acceptable social habit in the past. According to today's standard, smoking is categorized as an addiction.

Nicotine dependence occurs through smoking cigarettes, just as drug addiction occurs through substances like cannabis, cocaine and heroine.

Smoking these harmful substances becomes habitual and compulsive, and thus, an addiction develops. If the substance is withheld, withdrawal symptoms appear because the body has to re-adjust itself to function without the substance.

Research shows that most young smokers were influenced to begin the habit of smoking by their friends or older sibling. Advertising may reinforce the smoking habit. Media marketing techniques create the impression that smoking is a socially acceptable norm.

Smokers quickly become addicted to the nicotine in tobacco. When young people try to stop smoking, they experience similar withdrawal symptoms as adult smokers.

There are many negative health effects from smoking, such as coughs, increased phlegm, wheezing and shortness of breath. These problems start when an individual smokes his first cigarette. Also, there is the risk of dying prematurely from heart disease, lung cancer, and emphysema. Other effects experienced include accelerated osteoporosis, earlier menopause, and impaired reproductive capacity.

Cigarette smoking most likely will take hold during adolescence. Peer pressure is powerful and the popular crowd says," if you light up, you're cool with us." Young women think it's the thing to do because they look so elegant and worldly. When you inhale nicotine, the discharge of the dopamine is a pleasure hormone you experience immediately, and will give you immediate relief from tension.

When a pregnant woman smokes, her baby's brain development and birth weight is affected. Also, those babies have a higher risk of Sudden Infant Death Syndrome, (SIDS), hyperactivity, and behavioral problems. Chronic respiratory illnesses such as bronchitis, pneumonia and asthma are more common in infants and children who have one or both parents who smoke.

From the first moment a smoker rejects a cigarette, health benefits start to accrue. If an addicted smoker quits cold turkey, they may experience powerful withdrawal symptoms, which are physical and mental changes following interruption or termination of drug use.

When they stop smoking, many people experience symptoms like irritability, aggression, depressions, restlessness, poor concentration, increased appetite, light-headedness, waking at night and craving a cigarette. These symptoms generally last about two to four weeks.

Tips to Overcome Smoking

1. Nicotine replacement therapy such as chewing gum, skin patches, nasal sprays or inhalers ease withdrawal of the cravings and mood changes.
2. Bupropion (trade name Zyban) does not contain nicotine but can help an addicted smoker resist the urge to smoke
3. Accountability lends support. Do not try conquering your smoking addiction on your own. Enlist support of family and friends
4. Note habits or locations that are associated with smoking and change the routine
5. List reasons for freedom from smoking and read it when tempted to restart
6. Do not give up. Victory will come after a relapse. Try again and think what may have triggered the setback?

No quitting method will work unless you are genuinely committed to it and have some support. You will need a genuine desire to quit and lots of willpower.

The good news is that twenty minutes after quitting your heart rate will improve. After a few weeks, blood circulation improves, and cilia, (the tiny hair-like fibers in the lungs that remove mucus) grow back. Your risk of pancreatic and esophageal cancer drops.

LONG-TERM EFFECT OF SECOND HAND SMOKE:

A new study using a special type of MI shows visual evidence of exposure to second hand smoke over a period of time causes structural changes in the lungs of non-smokers.

The research was done at Children's Hospital of Philadelphia. Exposure was defined as living with a smoker for 10 years or more. Some of the non-smoking participants with extended exposure had holes and expanded spaces in their lungs just like the smokers. That type of damage is typical of emphysema. Second-hand smoke has been proven to affect individuals even when they never smoked, but had exposure to smoke. The risk of other cancers like kidney, cervical and brain cancer had increased. The most vulnerable are children. Mothers who smoke have increased risks for miscarriage, low birth weight, and infant stillbirths. Cigarette smoke is the leading cause of preventable death in the U.S.

On both public and private levels, the trend toward campus-wide smoking bans is proving to be effective. There are smoke-free campuses and many workplaces ban smoking and are smoke-free places. Some of the employees said they knew that smoke free areas were emerging, which gives them another reason to quit. Since smoke-free buildings and businesses were initiated, studies have shown higher productivity, fewer incidences of retirement for health reasons and lower health care costs. Work places have lower maintenance and cleaning costs, lower risks of fire and explosions as well as lower fire insurance premiums.

Nicotine addiction is defined as a chronic relapsing condition. Do not become frustrated by relapses. Many smokers will make multiple attempts to quit and it may take several attempts. Common reported reasons for relapse include stress, weight gain, depression and cravings. Relaxation techniques, weight management guidelines and continued support with pharmacological interventions are often the focus of these strategies.

WORKAHOLIC:

You love your work and are responsible for multiple projects and tasks.

Perhaps you own your own business and your hours are long. Vacations and social visits with friends are few. You don't spend much time with your family. Your only hobby is your job.

Workaholics live for their work, spending many hours at work, and often taking work home to complete. Americans compared to other nationalities typically work longer hours.

Because of down-sizing, consolidating and lack of replacement hiring, more workers are putting in extra hours to complete the work previously completed by others. Studies show that some workers do not take vacations or time off, because they fear they may lose their jobs.

Technological advances are part of the problem. We live and work in a connected environment; e-mails, instant messaging, fax machines, cell phones and digital assistants, make it hard to get time away from work.

Financial gain is determined by financial and materialistic measures, and that is how we mistakenly define success.

Regardless of the reasons, workaholism can be a serious condition that can lead to decline and destruction of families, as well as stress-related health problems. When this happens, it's time for intervention. Hard workers know the boundaries between work and personal time and can function normally when not at work. Workaholics have no personal time and cannot function outside of work.

Family and friends say you are working too much; putting in 12 to 14 hours at the office, working weekends and taking work home. This is a serious problem.

HOW TO TELL YOU ARE A WORKAHOLIC:

1. You feel compelled to work for the sake of working and feel panic or a sense of loss when not working
2. You feel loss, and unhappy without constant activity
3. Many of us know how to set boundaries. Occasionally we have to work long hours, but we have an internal regulator that tells us when we had enough
4. You regularly conceal from family members that you are working
5. You do not look for efficient or better ways to do things, but for ways to have more work to do
6. You get more excited about work than about family or other things
7. You take work with you on weekends and vacation

8. You like to talk about your work, and work more than 40 hours week
9. You turn your hobbies into money-making ventures
10. Your family and friends give up expecting you on time
11. You feel its okay to work long hours if you love what you are doing
12. You get impatient with people who have other priorities beside work
13. You are afraid that if you don't work hard, you will lose your job or be a failure
14. You constantly worry about the future even when things are going well
15. You do things energetically and competitively, including play
16. You get irritated when people ask you to stop doing your work to do something else
17. Your long hours disrupt your family life and other relationships
18. You think about your work while driving, falling asleep, or when others are talking
19. You work or read during meals
20. You believe that having more money will solve other problems in your life

Workaholics can put an enormous stress on co-workers if the workaholic is a manager. They would expect long hours from subordinates, might force them to meet impossible standards, then rush in to save the day when the work is substandard.

The workaholic may look like a hero, solving one crisis after another, when the crisis could have been avoided in the first place. Some workaholics have unwittingly created problems to provide an endless thrill of more work.

To bring balance back to your life, it will require some effort from you, your spouse, family and friends to shift from a sole focus on work. For the sake of your mental and physical well being, it is worth it.

MAKE TIME AWAY FROM WORK:

1. Set aside personal time to spend with family and friends (non work)

2. When traveling for business, call home regularly

3. Learn to delegate work and say" no" to new assignments

4. Do not volunteer for additional assignments. Take time off, starting with a long weekend

5. After clearing it with your doctor, consider an exercise routine. Enlist your spouse or friend as an exercise buddy

6. Consider volunteering in your community, helping others and meet new people

7. Convince yourself that it is okay to just sit and relax. Find a hobby.

8. Accept that we all need a decent number of hours of sleep

If you find difficult with any of these suggestions, consider getting professional help to deal with this addiction.

RELIGIOUS ADDICTION:

Inner Peace or Inner Turmoil

Religious beliefs are an important function in our daily lives and attitudes. Faith in God and adherence to religious rituals gives us moral guidance, emotional stability and valuable serenity.

However, fervent religious practices can signify other darker aspects of a person's mental health. For example, if someone's faith is used to mask or avoid psychological problems, or if their religious inclinations are taken to extremes, there is a possibility that the person is suffering from a psychiatric disorder. Too much religion may adversely affect people's social behavior, and their ability to function rationally.

Being religious is not an indication of bipolar or manic depressive behavior. A healthy approach to religious rituals is vital for the comfort and well being of people. It's a highly sensitive issue to question someone's beliefs or practices. Anything taken too far can do more harm than good. A term used to describe such a case is "hyper-religiosity".

In evaluating and assessing religiosity, consider some of the following:

1. Have they always been that way?
2. Does their zeal represent a sudden personality change?
3. Do the religious beliefs provide peace and personal contentment?
4. Has that person become belligerent and defensive?
5. Are they gentle in their speech or harsh, argumentative and self-righteous?
6. Have they become intolerant of other points of view?
7. Have people started avoiding them?
8. Has their quality of life improved or deteriorated?

Religion, like substance abuse can be a crutch. It can be an addiction. Just like any other addiction, religion may be used to hide other problems. Religion can be used as an addiction if it is used to conceal unresolved issues of shame, anger and authority.

Knowing what lies underneath that veneer of religion is critical to understand the hyper-religious person's behavior. It is important to know what brought about the change in attitude when someone's conspicuous preoccupation with religious belief and ritual takes on an extreme, consuming, new importance in their lives.

A Sudden Increased Interest In God and religion is often triggered by trauma or severe anxiety and may come in many forms:

1. Death of a loved one

2. A broken relationship
3. Serious illness or accident
4. Personal or financial loss
5. Incarceration

When security is threatened for whatever reason, people often turn to God. This is understandable; a confused, frightened individual who feels helpless will reach out for a source of comfort and solace. At what level does healthy, normal religious belief become abnormal?

One's ability to reason logically can become impaired. There is a tendency toward magical thinking that God will fix whatever the problem is without any serious work on your part. Confusion and doubts lead to mental, physical or emotional breakdown. One develops a fear-based belief system, believing and following a religion out of fear, not out of understanding and love. They also tend to have a shame-based belief system that they are not good enough or not doing anything right. They believe in a punishing and angry God.

Sincere faith in God is supposed to bring peace and contentment; A religious person who is paranoid and confrontational about it may have a larger mental problem. They tend to have increased conflict as well as an argumentative and defensive dialogue. They have a limited ability to explain their beliefs since their belief system about themselves is fear-based.

Hyper-Religiosity can be manifested as unusual self-importance such that the person mimics being much closer to God and others seem inferior. They develop judgmental attitudes and finds fault or evil in society. They tend to be blind to their own behaviors, denying their projections on to the idol "God" they have created.

Ritual is part of religion, but when it disrupts normal activities it is unhealthy. One is unable to function without unusually frequent rituals, rules, codes of ethics, or guidelines. Compulsive rituals or obsessive praying, quoting scriptures and excessive fasting often accompany the change in thinking patterns. Prayer and meditation are important aspects of faith, but they don't jeopardize a person's health or relationships.

Isolation and breakdown often follows. Detachment from work and relationships is noticeable as more and more time is spent in prayer and meditation. Manipulating scripture makes them feel specially chosen. They claim to receive messages from God. Thus, they move further away from the mainstream of social contacts.

They may also develop psychosomatic illnesses, back pains, sleeplessness, headaches, hypertension, etc. They are in denial of any personal problems. When behavior borders on manic or pathological, the hyper-religious person may start hallucinating, hearing voices, seeing images, or possibly "talking to God."

When an individual's interest in religion suddenly reaches a point of fixation, their regular lives are negatively affected; you could understand what is motivating their behavior. The problem could go away, but it also could get worse.

The believer assumes that their way to God is the only way. They become addicted to their faith. It becomes a means of escape. Instead of love of God softening their lives, it makes them harsh, rigid and limited.

WHEN RELIGION GOES BAD:

We may find it difficult to imagine that religion can ever go bad. Addiction substance alters our mood, and changes how we think and feel. Sometimes addictive substance alters our mood in ways that create undesirable feelings.

Preoccupation leads to a ritualized set of pre-acting out behavior. Like preoccupation, reutilization allows the addictive process to fill more time. This is true of addictions that do not involve consuming intoxicating substances. They fill days, even weeks with ritual preparations for acting out. We hurt people we care about. The result is guilt, shame and humiliation. This is a low state mood state.

Religious behavior can alter our mood. Like sex, food and work can alter our mood in positive ways, religious behaviors can alter our mood in positive, but it can also become a problem. Think about extreme examples such as religious suicide cult, or religiously motivated extreme self-deprivations or self-injury. Religious addiction is more common than you would conclude from looking only at the extreme cases. Addiction to religion is another addiction. God desires that we find a way to live without being addicted at all. The addictive cycle in religious addiction follows the same stages found in other addictions.

Specific behavior that is part of acting-out stage can vary. We may become obsessed with whether we have done well enough. You may leave church on Sunday to face the next week determined to live the Christian life, only to return the next week and hear that it wasn't good enough. Addictive religion never leads to soul rest. It leads to trying harder, which leaves us tired, frustrated and depressed.

At its root, religious addiction begins when faith stops being about a spiritual connection with God, and becomes an attempt to control our lives, or to control God by behaving in certain ways. These behaviors help us control our needs. Then they experience depression, a sense of meaninglessness or grief when they are not able to continue the behaviors. The behaviors interfere with our ability to maintain healthy relationships or function in life.

SHOPAHOLIC:

The stereotypical shopaholic darting from store to store to pick up anything and everything while racking up heavy credit card bills is not just stereotypical, but real life situations

There are some people who just buy what's on sale or what they need and nothing else. Then there are the compulsive shoppers who buy themselves into financial ruin.

The compulsive shopping is often viewed favorably rather than being treated as a problem.

Compulsive shoppers usually have low self-esteem, which appear to start as children. Children who experience parental neglect often grow up with low-self esteem throughout their childhood feeling like they are not important or wanted. As adults, they will depend on material things for emotional support, and likely to purchase anything in place of the toys they did not have as a child. Issues in their lives are repressed by buying something.

The credit cards, mail orders, catalogues and Internet facilitate the spending of money without leaving the house.

Like other addictions, shopping fills some kind of void. Compulsive buyers who took a twelve-step program called Debtors Anonymous also had certain personality types compared with the other addicts. They had low self-esteem, tendency toward fantasizing, depression and high anxiety.

It's not only women who become addicted to shopping. There are almost as many men. Women buy clothes, shoes, accessories, and jewelry while men are hooked on clothes, cars, gadgets, tools and electronics. The men are obsessed with auctions and are avid collectors of sport mementos, coins stamps and railroad trains.

Are You A Shopaholic:

1. Do you spend compulsively when you are feeling low?
2. Has your spending caused upset in your family or relationship?
3. Do you buy more than you planned on buying?
4. Do you buy items you don't need or clothes you don't wear?
5. Do you feel great when you are spending money?
6. Do you continue spending even though you are in debt?
7. Have you tried to stop unnecessary spending for any length of time?

Treatment is similar to other addictions. Look at your reasons for shopping, getting attention in a shop, novelty of buying something new. Do you feel something is missing? Are you drowning in debts?

1. Stop spending, cut up you credit cards, pay only in cash
2. Prioritize; pay off those with the highest interest rates first
3. Try to switch your debts to a lower rate of interest
4. If you have items in boxes that have never been used, return them or sell them online e-Bay or auctioning sites.
5. Work out a budget based on income and necessities. Buy only necessities and stick to your budget.

A shopaholic needs control, a guardian, and a certain credit limit. When in a store, the shopping takes precedence over everything and the addict will spend around two hours in a small store, looking for a sales.

Options for treatment can be individual or couples, counseling for compulsive buying Debtors Anonymous and Simplicity Circles.

Simplicity Circles can be a helpful support to shopaholics. They offer a place to gather with others to discuss transformation and satisfactions of living a simpler life. The caring atmosphere and the discussion of how to create a more fulfilling life is a healthy way to meet principal needs that a shopaholic seeks. It is the core and inner poverty, emotional and spiritual of most shopping addictions.

Women usually spend money on small items, such as clothing, jewelry, accessories etc. Men spend large amounts of money on cars and boats.

SHOPLIFTERS BATTLE WITH ADDICTION:

Shoplifters have their own technique that works for them. They would go to the store with a friend, and while the friend would take the clerk to get something away from the area of potential taking merchandise, the other person would grab what they wanted from the counter, put it in a bag or pocket, and go out of the store.

Some people steal an item and have a feeling of regret. Others repeatedly shoplift because it has become an addiction. Shoplifting addicts feel compelled to take things because they can easily grab what they want, and they get a rush of excitement from stealing. This makes the addict feel excited and energized because the risk of getting caught gives them a high.

Shoplifters come from a variety of backgrounds, some are rich, some are poor, but they all have low self-esteem. They believe they can't get in trouble, and usually get away with it; others feel they are entitled to have an item because it is owed to them. They feel that society owed it to them because their life was all screwed up.

Shoplifters think they will never get caught until they get busted. It is embarrassing to be marched through the mall in handcuffs, past friends and people you know. The embarrassment of the incident and the way people treat them after finding out they were shoplifting helped them stop.

Some addicts say that when they walk into a store, they feel the urge to take something. There will always be the excitement of wondering if they can still get away with it.

Shoplifters can cure their addiction by attending support groups and seeking therapy, not medication. Shopaholics must come to terms with themselves and their addiction in order to deal with the problem.

Some families train young children to be shoplifters, and they are taught to steal at a early age, and feel that is what to do. They feel good to just take whatever they want.

INTERNET ADDICTION:

There is a debate among users as to whether there really is such an addiction. It is a tool for gathering information, making new friends, and passing time.

Used in excess, the computer can become hazardous to one's mental and physical health.

The Internet provides an escape from reality and everyday problems. You can assume new identities, and interact with different people, It becomes a problem when people become engrossed and enmeshed in on-line activities to a point where they neglect their health, relationship and responsibilities.

The Internet allows for escape, love, knowledge, or just to have a lot of fun.

The World Wide Web is informative, convenient, resourceful, and fun.

<u>ARE YOU AN INTERNET ADDICT?</u> To be diagnosed, a person must meet certain criteria.

1. Tolerance, The need for increasing amounts of time on the Internet to achieve satisfaction

2. When reducing internet use, have two or more withdrawal symptoms such as tremors, anxiety, and obsessive thinking.
3. Use the Internet to relieve or avoid withdrawal symptoms
4. The Internet is accessed often, and for longer periods of time than intended
5. Spending a great amount of time in activities related to Internet use
6. Giving up important social, occupational or recreational activities to go on the Internet
7. Risk loss of relationship, job, educational, or opportunity because of excessive use of the Internet

Addictions vary according to sex, age, socioeconomic status, religion etc. and are most common in the middle socioeconomic classes.

The Internet is not the enemy just because people dependent on it. It is fast, convenient, and informative. It makes our lives simpler, and in ways, more complicated. It provides an escape from reality and everyday problems. People assume new identities, and find that the computer fills a social void.

Internet addiction can be harmful for those who dwell into the darker side of the web, such as online gambling, cybersex, and online affairs, online gaming, and pornography.

Both men and women "addicts" spent about the same amount of time online. Most said that chat room behavior on both parts interfered with important aspects of their lives.

The Internet invite's both genders to experiment in ways they might not do. I can't understand why people go online when they already have a sexual relationship and jeopardize their home, job, and lives.

Time alone cannot be an indicator of being addicted or having a compulsive behavior. For example, a college student will spend a great amount of time online doing research. A person with depression or social problems is more likely to spend time online because they don't want to be alone.

Usually, Internet addicts are likely newcomers to the Internet. They are going through the first stage of acclimating themselves to a new environment, and fully immersing themselves in it.

Once you admit you have a problem, or a disorder such as depression, see professional treatment for it. Once you admit and address the problem, other pieces of your life will fall into place.

Are you already addicted or tumbling toward trouble? The Internet Addiction Test is the validated reliable measure of addictive use of the internet, developed by Dr. Kimberly Young.

After you have answered all the questions, add the numbers of your responses to obtain your final score.

INTERNET ADDICTION TEST: To assess your level of addiction, think about the following questions, and answer them:

Rarely–1 point, Occasionally–2 points, Frequently– 3 points, Often–4 points, Always – 5 points

1. How often do you find that you stay on line longer then you wanted to
2. How often do you neglect household chores to spend more time on line
3. How often do you prefer the excitement of the internet to being with your partner
4. How often do you form new relationships with fellow on-line users
5. How often do others in your life complain to you about the amount of time you spend on-line
6. How often do your grades or school work, or job suffer because of the time you spend on-line
7. How often do you check your e-mail before doing something else that you want to do
8. How often does your job performance or productivity suffer because of the internet.
9. How often do you become defensive or secretive when anyone ask about what you do on line
10. How often do you block out disturbing thoughts about your life thoughts of the internet
11. How often do you find yourself anticipating when you will go on-line
12. How often do you fear that life without the Internet would be boring and joyless
13. How often do you snap, yell, or act annoyed if someone bother's you while you are on-line
14. How often do you lose sleep due to late-night log-ins

15. How often do you feel preoccupied with the internet when off, and fantasize about being on-line
16. How often do you find yourself saying "just a few more minutes on line
17. How often do you try to cut down the amount of time you spent on line and fail
18. How often do you try to hide how long you've been on-line
19. How often do you choose to spend more time on-line over going out
20. How often do you feel depresses, moody, or nervous when you are alone, which goes away once you are back on-line

20 – 49 points, you are an average on-line user
50 - 79 points, you are experiencing occasional or frequent problems
80 – 100 points, your Internet usage is causing significant problems. You should evaluate the impact of the Internet on your life and problems.

PLASTIC SURGERY:

Usually women think that a single plastic surgery is not enough to correct the appearance of their body. Many battle with a poor body image during puberty, and as they get older, will not accept their body as it is. They usually have an eating disorder, will not stick to diet and exercise, and opt for cosmetic surgery. They keep having surgery until they think their body is perfect. These are addicts who have an ideal outlook of what they want to look like. The lawmakers in California are pushing for stricter plastic surgery rules and regulations in the cosmetic surgery field.

Plastic surgery is not so negative as some people think, and it does have benefits. For example, children born with serious deformities may require plastic surgery to be accepted in society. Reconstructive surgery helps after major accidents where the occupants are severely disfigured or where a person cannot or will not live with a disfigurement. A 4-year-old boy had his chin rebuilt after a dog attacked him; a young women had a large birthmark on her forehead lightened with a laser. These are necessary plastic surgery procedures. Deformities are attention catchers and most people who have these feel inferior. In these cases, plastic surgery is essential. A person's appearance is the first thing you notice.

However, other beautiful and normal individuals choose to have plastic surgery. Many people experience plastic surgery for the first time and return again and again for more surgery. They return for more until they reach the excellent appearance and beauty they seek. Addiction to plastic surgery is known as body dysmorphic disorder. The individual sees themselves as hideous, regardless of how appealing they look.

Body bashing is counterproductive. Begin laying groundwork for a mature relationship with your body, and placing less emphasis on what you look like and more on how you feel. Women start to complain about their breasts being too small or too flat, lips too thin, hips too wide, nose too big, skin too dark or too light, hair too frizzy, arms too flabby, waist too thick etc. People want to change the size of their stomachs, breasts, or other body parts because they see it done so easily on TV turn to plastic surgery.

WHAT IS PLASTIC SURGERY :

The name is taken from the Greek work plastikos which means to form or mold. It is a special type of surgery that can involve a person's appearance and ability to function. Surgeons strive to improve patient's appearance and self-image through reconstructive and cosmetic procedures. This corrects defects on the face or body, such as physical birth defects, cleft lips and palates, ear deformities, traumatic injuries from bites or burns, and aftermath of diseases. Cosmetic procedures alter parts of the body the person is not satisfied with.

Teens view plastic surgery as a way to fit in and look acceptable to friends and peers. Adults see plastic surgery as a way to stand out from the crowd. Teens 18 and younger are having plastic surgery. Some people have plastic surgery to correct a physical defect or alter a part of the body that makes them feel uncomfortable. For example, guys with gynecomastia, a condition with excess breast tissue may opt for reduction surgery. Teens may have otoplasty surgery to pin back ears that stick out, or dermabrasion that smooth or camouflage severe acne scars. Most common procedures for teens are nose reshaping, ear surgery, acne and acne scar treatment.

Reconstructive surgery helps repair defects or problems, but to change your appearance is not a good idea. It will unlikely change your life. Plastic surgery is SURGERY, which involves anesthesia, wound healing, and other serious risks. Gastric bypass or liposuction may seem like quick and easy fixes compared to diets. People who are depressed have distorted views of what they look like and want to change their looks, thinking this will solve their problems. It won't. Many doctors will not perform plastic surgery if you are depressed or have other mental health problems until these problems are treated first.

In the last decade, cosmetic surgery has become as normal as having your hair done. Many have undergone various procedures, some stated it had improved their lives, some changed their jobs, and some changed their spouses.

The facelift is the most popular procedure in plastic surgery. Facelifts last about 10 years, and many patients repeat this procedure over and over again. The muscles are tightened and excess skin and fat are removed. This procedure is often performed with eyelid surgery, forehead lift, nose refinement or laser skin-resurfacing.

Plastic surgery is known as the "Career Tool". In Professor Gordon Patzer book, It is documented that good-looking people make more money than average looking, taller men make more than shorter men, and if a woman is just 13 lbs. overweight, she is penalized in some occupations. He states that looks do matter. We treat good looking people better. Salary discrepancy is true, even in law firms, where partner hiring seems to favor good-looking people. Even mothers treat good-looking babies and children better than average looking ones. Good looking attractive people earn, and make more money for companies.

Before everyone runs out to have plastic surgery, remember;

No regulations govern what type of medical practitioner can perform plastic surgery. American Society of Plastic Surgeons (ASPS) members are certified by the ASPS Board to perform plastic surgery of the face and all areas of the body; have 6 years of surgical training and experience with a minimum of 3 years of plastic surgery; operate only in accredited facilities; and fulfill continuing medical education requirements.

Many variables involve the pricing of plastic surgery, such as location, anesthesia, facility, fee etc.

Some plastic surgery is performed in non-accredited facilities.

Plastic surgery encompasses cosmetic and reconstructive surgery. ASPS members are trained, experienced, and qualified to perform all procedures on the face and all areas of the body.

Women mostly, and some men have a wax look, from skin tightly pulled over their face due to frequent plastic surgery.

RISKS AND COMPLICATIONS; (Every Surgery Carries Risk)

ANESTHESIA/SEDATION COMPLICATIONS - airway obstruction, blood clot, brain damage, heart attack, nerve damage, stroke, temporary paralysis

ASPIRATION - Vomiting during surgery, vomit is forced into the lungs

BLOOD LOSS – Excessive bleeding, drop in blood pressure

BLOOD CLOTS – Can be fatal. Pooling of blood

DROP IN BLOOD PRESSURE – Sudden drop due to blood loss

INFECTION – Antibiotics reduce this risk, longer surgery can lead to infection

LOOSE SUTURES – If the sutures come loose, this can lead to internal bleeding or hernia, and require additional surgery

COSMETIC SURGERY:

SKIN DEATH OR NECROSIS - Skin is surgically removed and may
affect the cosmetic outcome

ASYMMETRY – May require a second surgery. Moderate is normal

SLOW HEALING – Age, skin type, failure to follow doctor's orders

NUMBNESS/TINGLING – Temporary, sometimes permanent loss of
sensation. Injury to sensory motor nerves

IRREGULARITIES, DIMPLES, PUCKERS AND DIVOTS – due to
surgeon error or healing irregularities to body

SEROMA- Collection of fluid under the skin

GLOSSARY OF AESTHETIC PLASTIC SURGERY TERMS:

Abdominoplasty - (Tummy Tuck) Remove excess skin and fat

Alpha Hydroxy Acids - Removing layers of dead cells on skin

Augmentation Mammoplasty - (Breast Augmentation)

Blepharoplasty - (Eyelid Surgery)

Breast Augmentation – Enlarge small breasts or underdeveloped breasts

Breast Lift – (Mastopexy) Repositions breast tissue to a higher level and remove excess skin from lower portion.

Breast Implants – (Textured-Surface) Process creates a textured surface

Breast Reduction – Reduction Mammoplasty) Removing excess tissue

Buccal Fat Pad – Located above jaw line, & remove excessive fat. Gives A more contour look to face

Buttock Lift – Remove excess fat & loose skin and give a lift

Calf Augmentation – Implants to increase fullness of calf

Cannula – Hollow tub to remove fat layers under skin

Cellulite – dimpled looking fat surgically removed

Chemical Peel – Solution peels deeper layers of skin to remove wrinkles

Chin Augmentation - (Mentoplasty) Strengthen appearance of receding chin through incision inside of mouth

Collagen Injections – Injections to treat facial wrinkles

Dermabrasion – High speed rotary wheel used to abrade skin & acne

Earlobe Reduction – Earlobe reduction
Eyelid Surgery – (Blepharoplasty) Remove skin on eyelids

Facelift - (Rhytidectomy) Reduce sagging skin on face & neck
Fat Injections – Fat withdrawn from one body site injection into another
Forhead Lift – (Brow Lift) Improve skin wrinkling & sagging eyebrows

Hydroxyapatite Granules – Bone substitute made from coral used toenhance facial contours such as cheekbones

Labia – Surgery for vaginal tightening & labiaplasty re-shaping
Lasers – Eliminate surface blood vessels on the face
Lip Augmentation – Surgically advancing the lip forward & injecting fat
Lip Lift – Surgically lifts corners of aging mouth
Lip Reduction – A strip of the mucosa is surgically removed
Lipoplaty – (Liposuction) Removes collections of fatty tissue from the Abdomen, buttocks, legs, back, arms, face & neck

Malar - (Cheekbone) Augmentation Cheekbone built up by placing an Implant over them through an incision in the mouth

Otoplasty – (Ear Surgery) Reshaping the cartilage behind the ear

Peel –(Buffered Phenol)   Formula for severely sun-damaged skin

Phenol – Chemical used for full face peeling from sun damage and wrinkles around the mouth.

Rhinoplasty – (Nose Reshaping) To alter the size and shape of the nose

Sex Change Surgery - Reassignment, reconstructive, and cosmetic surgery.

Tattooing - (Cosmetic) Micro pigmentation, for permanent eyeliner
                eyebrows, lip color, blush and eye shadow. Used to recreating the colora areola around the nipples

TCA – Trichloroacetic acid for peeling of the face, neck, hands etc.
                It has less bleaching effect and is excellent for peeling of specific areas. Used for deep, medium or light peeling

TANNING BEDS:

Tanning beds and salons are the latest in fashion for the young people today. Teens and young adults today are using tanning beds as a way to have that year round tan. Going to the prom or dances now include not only getting your hair and nails done but also going to the tanning beds, even if you live down south or near the beach. It's fashionable to have that natural looking sunless tan all year. They mistakenly think they can tan without the harmful effects of the sun, sand, or peeling. You can pick the shade of tan, accent flattering features and have a healthy natural glow in about 15 minutes. Bronze, artificial tanning, airbrush tanning, fake tans, tanning lotions body mists and sprays are just some of the sunless tans available today. You pick the shades, how light or dark you want to be, and in the comfort of the tanning bed. Airbrush and spray use a non toxic sugar, (DHA) Dihydroxyacetone, sprayed 1-20 minutes and last about 5 to 7 days

People with limited time to spend in the sun want to tan in private, or want just a certain shade of tan will go to tanning salons or booths.

Tanning salons give clients protective goggles to protect their eyes, and people prone to sunburn let staff at the tanning salons know about how much sun they can take.

TANNERS COULD BECOME ADDICTED ON UV RAYS:

In a 2006 study, researchers at Wake Forest University may have solved the question as to why many men and women who obsessively tan, may have an addiction to the UV rays of tanning beds.

The remedy for natural gloom of winter is a visit to a tanning salon. There is a lure to tanning beds, despite the cancer warning. Studies on tanning beds use say tanners experience withdrawal symptoms. When chemicals stimulate the skin by exposure to UV rays, there is a feeling of relaxation.

If you feel bad when you cannot tan, you may be a tanning addict.

Those who tanned frequently were more apt to UV rays based tanning beds than their less tanning counterparts. When the skin gets darker from tanning, it is actually a product of skin cell damage. Tanning beds are no safer than directly tanning in the sun.

Tanning dermatologists have found that during tanning, the skin give off endorphins. These opioid compounds make a person feel good. Frequent tanning may be a type of substance abuse. Studies done by Dr. Richard Wagner Jr. and Dr. Kaur suspected that frequent tanners get hooked on the endorphins produced by tanning under ultraviolet light. The skin makes endorphins when it's exposed to UV light, the same light that causes skin cancer. Three types of skin cancer are; basal cell carcinoma, squamous cell care, and most serious, melanoma. Even this information does not deter tanners.

A tanning addict usually has an unlimited pass to a tanning salon and goes 8 or more times a month. They say tanning beds are safe, but there is no such thing as safe tanning. Tanning makes them feel relax and happy. Most teens between the age of 14 and 17 start tanning at this early age.

Frequent tanners get withdrawal symptoms when given naltrexone, a drug that blocks a narcotic-like substance produced in the skin during tanning. The frequent tanners reported being nausea or jitteriness.

According to the American Academy of Dermatology, tanning booth exposure can cause cataracts and eye damage, premature aging of the skin and skin cancer.

Self-Confessed TanAholic.:
This 34 year old mom visits a tanning booth 3 times a week. States she cannot live without the beauty of the bronzed look and that she looks sickly without her base tan. Her skin looks terrible, loose and wrinkled, mottied-color and leathery looking. When she was asked why she is doing this to herself, she said it makes her feel so good.

In the study, frequent tanners were given a drug that blocked the pleasurable sensations that went along with the tanning-bed experience. After their sessions, half of them suffered withdrawals. They complained of nauseous, jittery, and sick to their stomach. Those using UV tanning beds were more relaxed and happy than those who did not.

ADDICTION: You heard people say, "Just quit already," It's easier to talk about it than to do it. Process of becoming addicted is easy, but to stop is extremely difficult, but not impossible.

How to start? Where do you go? Ask your physician, or call your local hospital, and they will direct you, step by step.

You will not be alone. You will have support service, individual counseling, family and support groups.

When you think of an addict, you think of a person with a habit so strong that he or she cannot easily give it up. It does not say impossible, but that it will take time, and will be difficult, but NOT IMPOSSIBLE.

TELEVISION ADDICTION:

Do you have a compulsion to watch television all the time? Television addiction is like drugs or alcohol, etc. in the manner that it alters the mental state of the subject.

For decades, television viewing has been studied, and there still is not an accepted checklist in diagnosing the addiction. However, it is a problem faced by many people.

It affects the lives of people because the person does not accomplish anything, but has this uncontrollable compulsion to continue watching anything and everything. They neglect their house, family; experience a lack of motivation, feelings of anger, depression and listlessness. When the person tries to go for long periods of time without watching TV, they often feel withdrawal symptoms and anxiety.

The average person spends about three to five hours a day watching TV. Some heavy viewers spent about eight hours a day in front of the boob tube.

Would you call them addicted to TV? Would you consider this an unusually large amount of time?

ARE YOU ADDICTED?

Addiction is spending an unusually large amount of time watching TV.

1. When you arise in the morning, do you put on the TV while eating breakfast or having coffee?
2. If on the job, the office or booth, do you have the TV on all day?
3. During lunch, or in a business waiting room, do you sit near the TV?
4. Do you have a TV in the bathroom, or on your small boat?
5. Do you eat your meals, (lunch and dinner) in front of the TV?
6. Do you stay home; have no social life because you want to watch TV.

Today, everywhere you go, there is a TV set. The stores, gym, medical offices, bank, repair shops, garages, airports, airplanes, etc. It's difficult to escape.

Addiction is spending more time in front of the TV than intended and having unsuccessful attempts to stop. TV is for relaxation, entertainment, and distraction, yet, when some people attempt to reduce TV viewing, they are unable to do so. When they do succeed, they report withdrawal symptoms. In Japan, it is reported that children were treated for epileptic seizures that was attributed to a program called "Pokemon" that flashed colorful lights.

Laboratory experiments done on people's reactions to TV were done by monitoring brain waves via an electroencephalograph. The studies showed less mental stimulation measured by alpha brain wave production during watching TV. The TV had a numbing effect, and the body relaxed as if it was tranquilized. Drowsiness occurred, and depression set in. The person watching TV became disengaged in reality and became immersed and part of what was on the TV.

TV allows the person to blot out the real world and enter into a world of make believe, a pleasurable and passive mental state. You no longer have the worries and anxieties of reality, and you become absorbed in a TV program by going on a "trip", induced by the TV. People overestimate their control over TV watching, put off other activities to spend hours watching TV. When the TV is on, they resume living in a different, less passive style.

Heavy viewers find the TV irresistible, and cannot ignore it. They state they cannot turn it off, that as they reach out to turn the TV set off; the strength goes out of their arms. So, they sit for hours and watch it.

TV addicts state they know they have things to do, but cannot do them, such as plant the garden, cut the grass, sew, crochet, do some crafts, play games, take the baby out for fresh air, take walks with their spouse, etc. The house is no longer clean, laundry remains undone, and meals are not cooked. Medical and dentist appointments are no longer kept. These activities are no longer desirable, and they must watch TV. They have passed up the activities that lead to growth and development.

Adverse effect of TV distorts the sense of time, and renders other experiences vague and unreal. It weakens relationships by reducing and eliminating normal opportunities for talking and communicating. The family is no longer communicating and drifting apart.

To avoid addiction,

Keep a record of how much time is spent on TV watching,
1. List what you could be doing at home instead of watching TV,
2. Keep the list of things you should be doing instead of watching TV,
3. Have a list of household projects you want to do or complete. such as outside activities, reading, sports etc.
5. Limit how much you can watch in a day, a week, etc., and stick to it.
6. Consider exercising while watching TV, such as a stationary bike, treadmill etc.

Violence and objectionable material on TV has become worse and worse.

Some families are getting rid of their TV due to the caliber of the subject matter on TV. They feel that TV has hijacked their family, and want family meetings, family meals, family conversation etc. back. They state that they now have a healthy relationship, and time for their family that was robbed by the TV. They protected their children and showed the children that they meant more to the parents than TV. They protected their family from TV addiction. When the family was interviewed, they all stated that giving up the TV was the best solution for them. Get some guidelines and stick to your commitment.

VIDEO GAME ADDICTION;

Video game overuse is also known as video game addiction, which is known as a form of psychological addiction. It's the use of a computer and video games. Instances have been reported where the users play compulsively, isolating themselves, and focusing entirely on the game, not normal life events.

The American Medical Association is still discussing the topic, and need further research before video game addiction could be a formal diagnosis.

Symptoms of video game addiction are similar to other psychological addictions, like compulsive behavior and impulse control disorder. Symptoms of impulse control disorder include regular displays of compulsion, loss of control, and withdrawal when prevented from playing. The player may commit illegal acts to sustain the activity, despite any adverse consequences. Also, some rely on others to finance their activities.

1. Preoccupation and consistent playing of the video game
2. Unable to stop or control the game
3. Telling lies to friends & family about the extent of the activity when playing the game
4. Irritability and restlessness when prevented from playing the game

5. Increasing time spent on the game to satisfy or achieve goals for the game, and needs to spend more and more time on the activity.

Video game overuse or addiction is common in other countries, such as Asia and South Korea and most common in ages 9 to 39.

A survey done by the Entertainment Software Association found that video game overuse was more common in players of MMORPG. An interview done by Dr. Maressa Orzack of McLean Hospital in Belmont Mass. estimated that 40% of the million players of MMORPG World of Warcraft are addicted.

Men may be more prevalent than women when the games revolve around territorial control. The part of the brain that generates rewarding feeling is more activated in men than in women when they play video games. It appears that playing video games can satisfy some basic psychological needs of men, and they want to continue to play because of the rewards, freedom and a connection with other players.

Addiction to computer games may be caused by psychological problems, antisocial personality disorder, depression and social phobias. Many addicts see this as a way to escape reality and find that they can create a new persona with online games and live their life through this new online personality. It starts out as a fantasy life, more than reality due to newfound friends and power, and many refuse to be drawn away from it. This is seen as an addiction and needs to be treated on the same level as an addiction. There is a lot of controversy over video game addiction being diagnosed as a disease.

China and South Korea have treated video games as an addiction, and limited the number of hours teenagers can spend online playing games. After three hours, players under 18 are prompted to stop.

As with other addictions, the most effective treatments are a combination of psychopharmacology, psychotherapy and twelve-step, self-help, support and recovery organization for gamers.

VIEWS ON ADDICTION TODAY

More and more technology is coming into our lives to serve man in industry, commerce, medicine and other fields. The public utilizes all these wonderful technical equipment and knowledge that is available, and it is very difficult to do without. No wonder we are all moving toward being addicted to all the comforts and technology that is available.

We face critical choices about how to view and attack addiction. Addiction is the symptomatic malady of our society today.

The conventional view of addiction does nothing except convince people of their vulnerability. It is one more element in a pervasive sense of loss of control that is the contributor to all substance abuse and addiction. It is important to rationalize the cost of self respect and family values that result from the loss of control the addict is experiencing. Science cannot increase our understanding of our world and ourselves. The bottom line is that the addict must be in control, and take the initiative for his or her life and future. They must decide what is more important; their lives, health, future, family, friends, and job, or their demons, the addiction.

Addiction can be overcome, and it will not be easy. The results will be up to the addict as to what is more important to them. It is a battle worth fighting for, and you can win. Others have done it, and so can you. You can have a future, a life without addiction.

There is nothing you cannot do if you put your mind to it

If something is easy to do, it can be accomplished immediately,

If something is hard to do, you must work at it,

If something is impossible to do, it can be done, but it will take a little longer.

There is nothing you cannot do, or be, if you set your mind to it. We are different from animals because we have a choice as to what we want to do, and the decisions we make. We are free to make that choice. We may make mistakes, but nothing is written in stone. We can change it.

SUMMARY: You are in control of your own life. Your body is your temple, you want to keep it clean and healthy; no garbage should be put in your body such as alcohol, drugs, and any other substance abuse. When you abuse any substance, you are no longer in control of your body, and the demons take over, with their cruel torture, racking your body in pain. There is an old saying," garbage in, garbage out." When you give in, and continue to take the abusive substance to take away the pain, the devil has won. He wants your soul. You have everything to LOSE. Nothing to GAIN.

When you resist, and it's not easy, God is on your side, with the help of your family, friends, and community organizations. Remember that God made you, and he does not make junk. You are precious, and God is here to help you if you let him. Your future is up to you. The ball is in your court. You can do it. We are your cheering section. Everyone is on your side. You have nothing to lose, and everything to gain. Your life and your future are the prize to be won.

Addiction is like an Boa Constrictor snake. It coils around your body; its slimy body crushes your body, tighter and tighter until you no longer are capable of breathing, and the snake has won. You can beat your addiction and win your battle. Do not allow yourself to lose control, the snakes takes over, and you are helpless. You can still fight, you are still boss of your body, your temple. Do not give in to the snake. Keep your body clean. Remember, you only have one body, and, do not give it up.

Take control, be proud, work toward your life and future.

WARNING SIGNS TO TAKE NOTICE AND ACTION;

Alcohol Abuse:
Availability of alcohol is priority at all functions
and activities
Changes in skin appearance, flushed skin
Chronic lateness
Frequent medical leaves
Frequent shaking and trembling,
especially in the morning
Frequent trips to medical providers
General tacky unkempt appearance
Increase or decrease in weight
Individual is erratic, irritable, difficult to get along with
Legal difficulties
Medical leave of several days duration
Misses work on Mondays and Fridays
Misses deadlines and assignments
Needs a drink to relieve stress
Odor of alcohol around the individual
Poor judgment
Quality of presentations deteriorates
Quality of work deteriorates
Quickly drinks several drinks
Repeated complaints of lack of energy, headache etc
Repeated bruises and scrapes
Trouble with decision making

Drug Abuse:
Aggressive or social with-drawl

Appears intoxicated or hung over
Confused and indecisiveness
Distrustful and suspicious
Forgetfulness, short attention span
Frequent absence and unknown where individual is
Frequent medical visits
Loses touch with reality
Loss of mental sharpness

Inability to control emotions, overreacting
No sense of humor
Overall attitude changes
Physical appearance and grooming deteriorating
Unpredictability, inappropriate behavior
Withdrawal from responsibility

Stimulants:
Stimulants include: acid, amphetamines, cigarettes, coaine, crack, crystal meth, desoxyephedrine, ecstasy, freebase, hallucinogens, LSD, nicotine, pseudoephedrine, methamphetamine, magic mushrooms, MDMA, psilocybianc, club drugs etc.

Behavior
Chronic financial difficulties even with
an adequate income
Compulsive cleaning, sorting, etc.
Dry mouth and nose, teeth grinding, body tremors
Euphoria, expansive mood
False sense of confidence
Increased physical activity
Irritable, argumentative, nervous

Progressive violent or aggressive behavior
Purposeless, repetitious behavior
Runny nose, cold or chronic sinus infections
Talkative, excited speech
Use or possession of drug paraphernalia including spoons, razor, powder

Depressants:
Depressants include: ativan, barbiturates, codeine, lorazepam, muscle relaxants, etc.
Behaves as if drunk
Flaccid appearance
Flat affect
Slurred speech

Opiates:
Opiates include: buprenorphine, codeine, coricidin, darvocet, heroin, lotab, hydrocodone, morphine, norco, opioids oxycontin, oxycodone, prescription painkillers, (scrips) suboxone, vicodan etc.
Euphoria, tranquility, impaired judgement
Excessive active, frantic, or lethargic drowsy
Frequent itching and scratching
Nausea
Red and raw nostrils from sniffing
Slow breathing
Wears long sleeves even when not injecting needles

RESOURCES / REFRENCES:

Many sources of information has been utilized during research of this book; such as computer information and websites, books, newspapers, magazines, articles in various publications, interviews, and especially my personal experience in the hospital setting with addicts. It was written to help individuals "kick" their addiction, and encourage them not to give up, and hang in there. They can do it.

Many thanks to the resources and references, which validate authentication of this book, and the people who freely gave me information. I want to give credit to everyone who contributed any information, regardless how small it was. Thank you, thank you, and thank you! They are all sincerely appreciated.

Bartscherer, Diane; R.N., M.S. ANP-C
Becky, Worley
Bellantoni, Michele, M.D.
Benson, April Lane; Psychologist, N.Y.
Belluck, Pam; Net Addiction; 1996
Bratter and Forest, 1985
Brodland, Gene; Professor, South Illinois University
Brody, Dr., American Academy of Child & Adol. Psychiatry
Bryner, Jeanna; March, 2008
Burton, Tara
Carter, Molly
Cooper

Copper Devlin, Null, Christopher, Ben Patterson, Robin
    Raskin
Custer, Robert;   MD
Cutter, Deborah;   Psychiatrist
Diaz, Virginia, Henando Today
Durand, Jacobs; Ph.D.
Edginton, Thomas; Dr.
    Edwards, Drew W; M.S.
Edwards, Elizabeth; Eastern Michigan University
Egger and Rauterberg; 1999

Ellis, Christensen, Tricia
Elliott, Lyndsay
Erickson, Patricia; Nursing Coordinator
Fassel, Diane
Fernandez, Belkys
Ferris, Jennifer; Ph.D.
Folan, Patricia; R.N., BSN
Freeman; 1992
Gebhardt, Scott; Dr.
Getzenberg, Robert; M.D.
Gluckman, Dr.
Gold, Mark, M.D.
Goldberg, Ivan; MD, Psychiatrist
Grohol, John M., Psychiatrist, 1997
Hansen, Randall; Ph.D.
Hauptman, Manuel
Herbert, Josef; Associaated Press
Herkov, Michael;   Ph.D., 2006
Higgins, Dilara
Hillyard, Pam; Manager
Homes, Leonard; Ph.D.

Hughes, Gina
Jacobsel, Dan; R.N., BSN
Jaffe-Gill, Ellen, M.A.
Kaur, Mandeep, Md., Dermatologist
Koran, Lorrin, Dr; Stanford University Psy.
Korkki, Phyllis
LavaMind, 1997
Lee, Michelle; Capt. Kent Police
Lesieur, Henry, Ph.D.
Lopez, Luis; Tampa Tribune
Luft, Robert and Mary Rose
Lunn, Emma
Manolls, Chris; XAVIER University, Ohio
Mazhar Uzma; 2000
McCall, Karen; Counseling, Financial Recovery

McElroy and Goldsmith
McGraw, Randee; Adm. Director
Moore, Coleen; Coordinator of Resource Development
Mostwin, Jacek L.
Orzack, Maressa, Dr.McLean Hospital, Belmont, Mass.
Peele, Stanton, Ph.D., J.D.

Rauterberg, M. Egger; 1996
Reyno, R.L.
Roberts, James; Baylor University, Texas
Roberts, Smith and Pollack, 1996
Robinson, Ann; Consumer Policy at U Switch
Robinson, Bryan, Psychotherapist, North Carolina
Robinson, Evan, Music & Choir Director
Rowe, Dorothy, Psychiatrist
Ryan, Dale

Ryan, Richard, Univ. of Rochester & Immersyve Inc.

Segal, Jeanne; Ph.D.
Segal, Robert; M.A.
Shapiro, Kenneth, MD
Shapiro, Valerie
Skinner, B.F.; Operant Conditionial
South Shore Skin Center, Massachuset
Stengle, Jamie; The Associated Press
Stryker, Jeff, 2000
Suler, John; Ph.D
Van Vonderen, Jeff
Wagner, Richard Jr., MD, Dermantology
Walters, John P.
Weathers, Laura; MD, Tribune Correspondent
Wikipedia, the free encyclopedia
Winn, Marie, The plug-in drug
Young, Kimberly; Ph.D.
Zehr, Rick, V.P, of Addiction & Behavior Sciences

ORGANIZATIONS

Addiction Treatment
Alcohol Addiction
All About Life Challenges
American Council for Drug Education
American Heart Association
Behavioral Medicine Associates
Bromenn Regional Medical Center, Illinois
Canerbury Institute
Center for Online Addiction

Children, Youth & Women's Health Services, So, Australia

Cancer Society

Comprehensive Modern Mental Health Services
Drug Addiction

Ellis, Ann-Gayle; Hernando County

Health Information Publications, 2002-2005

Illinois Institute for Addiction Recovery, Springfield

International Service Organization of SAA, Inc.

Internet Addiction Test. Center for Internet Addiction Recovery

JAMA

John Hopkins Medicine

Mayo Clinic Health / Library

National Council on Alcoholism & Drug Education

National Institute on Drug Abuse

PBS On Line

Proctor Hospital, Peoria, Illinois

Realization Center Food Addiction Program

Schick Shadel Hospital

Smoking Addiction and Nicotine Addition

Teens Health

The Partnership for a Drug Free America

University of Utah

U.S. Food & Drug Administration

Drug and Alcohol Treatment Centers